GUIDE TO EDUCATION

Guide to Education and Training for Primary Care

Edited by
YVONNE CARTER and NEIL JACKSON

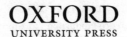

OXFORD
UNIVERSITY PRESS

OXFORD

UNIVERSITY PRESS

Great Clarendon Street, Oxford OX2 6DP

Oxford University Press is a department of the University of Oxford.
It furthers the University's objective of excellence in research, scholarship,
and education by publishing worldwide in

Oxford New York

Athens Auckland Bangkok Bogotá Buenos Aires Cape Town
Chennai Dar es Salaam Delhi Florence Hong Kong Istanbul Karachi
Kolkata Kuala Lumpur Madrid Melbourne Mexico City Mumbai Nairobi
Paris São Paulo Shanghai Singapore Taipei Tokyo Toronto Warsaw
with associated companies in Berlin Ibadan

Oxford is a registered trade mark of Oxford University Press
in the UK and in certain other countries

Published in the United States
by Oxford University Press Inc., New York

© Oxford University Press, 2002

The moral rights of the authors have been asserted
Database right Oxford University Press (maker)

First published 2002

A catalogue record for this title is available from the British Library

Library of Congress Cataloging in Publication Data

Guide to education and training for primary care / edited by
Yvonne Carter and Neil Jackson.
Includes bibliographical references and index.
1. Primary care (Medicine)–Study and teaching–Great Britain.
I. Carter, Yvonne, 1959- II. Jackson, Neil.
[DNLM: 1. Physicians, Family–education–Great Britain. 2. Education,
Medical–Great Britain. 3. Primary Health Care–Great Britain.
W 18 G9457 2001]
R772.G85 2001 610′.71′141–dc21 2001036738

1 3 5 7 9 10 8 6 4 2

ISBN 0 19 263293 0

Typeset by Florence Production Ltd, Stoodleigh, Devon
Printed in Great Britain
on acid-free paper by
Biddles Ltd., Guildford & King's Lynn

Contents

List of contributors

Michael Bannon, Associate Dean of Postgraduate Medicine, London Deanery, University of London

Reed Bowden, Associate Dean of Postgraduate General Practice, London Deanery, University of London

Jonathon Burton, Associate Dean of Postgraduate General Practice, London Deanery, University of London

Yvonne Carter, OBE, Professor of General Practice and Primary Care, Queen Mary, University of London

Charles Easmon, Director of Workforce Development, NHS Executive London

Maggie Falshaw, Research Manager, Department of General Practice and Primary Care, Queen Mary, University of London

Rosslynne Freeman, Professor of Educational Development in Medicine, Aga Khan University, Karachi

Amanda Howe, Professor of Primary Care, University of East Anglia

Sir Donald Irvine, CBE, President, General Medical Council

Neil Jackson, Dean of Postgraduate General Practice, London Deanery, University of London

Alex Jamieson, Associate Dean of Postgraduate General Practice, London Deanery, University of London

Neil Johnson, Postgraduate Dean, NHS Executive Trent and University of Leicester

Comfort Osonnaya, Chadburn Fellow, Department of General Practice and Primary Care, Queen Mary, University of London

Elisabeth Paice, Dean Director of Postgraduate Medicine, London Deanery, University of London

David Percy, Director of Workforce Development, NHS Executive South East

Helen Prentice, Lead Nurse for Young People and Womens' Health, Epping Forest PCT

Mike Pringle, Chairman, Royal College of General Practitioners

Tony Rennison, Associate Dean of Postgraduate General Practice, London Deanery, University of London

John Schofield, Associate Dean of Postgraduate General Practice, London Deanery, University of London

Dame Lesley Southgate, President, Royal College of General Practitioners

John Spencer, Professor of Medical Education in Primary Health Care, University of Newcastle upon Tyne

Tony Weight, Deputy Director of Workforce Development, NHS Executive London

Patricia Wilkie, Chairman, Lay Advisory Panel, College of Optometrists

Foreword

SIR DONALD IRVINE CBE

For patients, good quality primary health care is of fundamental importance. Primary care is the service to which we first turn when we become ill. It is our general practitioners and nurses who support and sustain us through chronic illness and who care for us when medical science has nothing more to offer. And we rely on them primarily for our preventive health care.

Primary health care has survived in the distinctive form we know today because, in the main, it has provided patients with a quality of health care which they appreciate and value. It is the part of the NHS people know best. Patients relate their perceptions of quality to individual health-care professionals – the family doctor, the practice nurse, the receptionist – rather than to a much more nebulous institution – such as the hospital. People talk about 'their practice'. Quality begets trust. It stems from the belief that the doctor, nurse, or receptionist is acting with patients' best interests as their only objective. So for patients, quality in relation to their practice is a very personal thing.

Quality, and the trust that is built up through it, consists of an amalgam of several ingredients. Technical competence is vital. Doctors and nurses must know what they are doing. They have a duty to keep themselves thoroughly up to date and effective in their chosen field. Attitudes and interpersonal skills are equally important.

Doctors and nurses have to be good communicators and
be empathetic, respectful, and caring. Equally they must
be honest, open, and truthful – integrity is a core ingredient of trust.

Then there is the environment for care – another
element of quality. Is the surgery warm, comfortable, wel-
coming? Is access easy? Are there systems in place to
support quality practice, for example good records and the
data systems needed to inform audit and risk management? Last but not least, there is the all-important matter
of time. Has the primary care group or trust created the
time essential for doctors and nurses to be able to give
good personal patient care, and for professional development and the regular quality assurance of their practice?

In terms of quality, I regard the education and continuing professional development of members of the practice
team as a high priority. Good education and training,
informed by regular feedback through the results of practice quality assurance, is what is most likely to keep everyone at the cutting edge. Successful primary care groups
and trusts will show their understanding of the importance of this by the extent to which they invest time,
money, and effort in making it possible for all their health
professionals to take part and benefit to the fullest possible
extent.

Hence the importance and timeliness of this book.
Yvonne Carter and Neil Jackson have brought together a
group of well-known practitioners to help them give an
up-to-date and comprehensive account of education and
training for primary care. They succeed well. Readers will
find much in here which will help them chart the way
forward in their own practice teams in ways that should
lead to good results for patients and that enhanced professionalism in practitioners so crucial to their satisfaction
and morale.

Introduction

YVONNE CARTER AND NEIL JACKSON

Quality in general practice and the wider context of primary care can only be achieved by a system of service development and delivery which is supported and informed by the systems of education and training and research and development, i.e. a 'three-systems approach'.[1]

With the advent of primary care groups and primary care trusts (PCGs/PCTs) and a huge government programme of primary care development comes a greater need to understand the education and training system and its role in the NHS. This handbook will also seek to encourage and facilitate strategic thinking and planning in relation to education and training at various levels including organizational, team, and individual health-care professional.

A primary care strategy for education and training should include the following key elements:

- PCGs/PCTs will need to build in a clear education and training agenda to their developmental programmes, which should include an understanding of workforce planning and multiprofessional/multidisciplinary skill mix and the implications for professional revalidation and regular peer appraisal.
- Effective leadership for education and training in primary care must be established which is linked to clinical governance and quality health care.

- The various education and training funding schemes must be understood in order to take full advantage of available financial resources.
- Learning and development must occur at various levels in the primary care setting, i.e. PCGs/PCTs, staff in practices, and the community.
- Personal learning and development should be linked to practice organization, learning, and development, i.e. the concept of personal development plans (PDPs) linked to practice professional development plans (PPDs).
- Learning will need to take place across professional and organizational boundaries, e.g. across the primary and secondary care sectors in the NHS.
- Promoting a greater understanding of the roles of existing and future educational organizations/structures and their educational networks, e.g. undergraduate/ postgraduate departments of general practice, new workforce development confederations, and higher education institutions.
- Developing the concept of fitness for purpose. Although fitness for practise remains of crucial importance for all primary care health-care professionals, whether medical or non-medical, the concept of fitness for purpose is now paramount. This implies that there is a need for a highly skilled and integrated multidisciplinary workforce of health-care professionals who must work and learn together to deliver the future primary care agenda.

It is intended that the readership of this handbook should extend to primary health-care professionals and organizations, including health authorities and primary care groups/trusts, medical and non-medical undergraduate and postgraduate students; health-care professionals, and organizations in the secondary care sector including acute and mental health trusts; other relevant NHS organizations, e.g. NHS(E) regional offices, patients, and lay members of the public.

In order to continue to improve services and develop confidence in the delivery of high-quality health care, GPs, primary health-care teams, and hospital doctors need to monitor the care they provide and audit their experience and practice against standards and examples of good practice. We hope that the inclusion of chapters on audit, primary/secondary care interface issues, and learning from patients will facilitate this.

It is also hoped that this book will act as a useful reference guide to countries outside the United Kingdom with developing health-care systems, some of which are based on UK models of primary care.

In background, the two editors of this book are both experienced teachers of both undergraduates and postgraduates and have demonstrated a commitment to multi-professional education and training. Perhaps more importantly, we are experienced in day-to-day clinical care in the community and at the interface with secondary care. This book has gathered together what we consider to be an impressive array of contributors with a wide variety of experience. We hope that the handbook conveys the excitement and enthusiasm each contributor feels for their subject, and will, we hope, provide both theoretical and practical guidance for those delivering and receiving education and training in an ever-changing primary care setting.

The editors would like to acknowledge their thanks to Sir Donald Irvine for writing the foreword, to the co-authors for their excellent contributions, to Olivette Stanislas for all her administrative support and to the commissioning editor, Helen Liepman, for her patience and

professional guidance in the preparation and development
of this book.

References

1. Jackson N. Quality in the new NHS – the role of education and train-
    ing in general practice and primary care. *Education for General Practice*
    1999; **10**: 6–8.

1 Education and training in the NHS in England

DAVID PERCY AND CHARLES EASMON

Introduction

The organization and funding of education and training systems within the NHS in England is complex and difficult to understand. This is largely because it results from the bringing together over the years of a number of differing systems without any attempt in the past to make sense of the whole rather than the individual parts. At the time of writing this failing is starting to be tackled, although this process will itself take a little while. Along with an appreciation of the need for the different disciplines that work together to learn together, where appropriate, so that they can better understand their different roles, the importance of seeing education and training as a whole system, linked with research and supporting and informing service delivery, is finally being widely recognized. Education and training is a means to an end, that of providing good quality health care, not an end in itself.

The organization and funding of education and training for clinical professionals in the NHS began to take shape in the late 1980s with the publication of *Working for Patients*[1] and the 11 working papers that accompanied it. The tenth, now often just referred to as working paper 10, covered the education and training of the main professional groups other than doctors and dentists. It established some key principles:

- first, the education of these groups should move from health service control with the existing colleges of nursing, health, etc., which were closely identified with local NHS institutions, not the higher education sector.
- second, that the NHS led by the regional health authorities should agree contracts with higher education for the provision of basic qualifying education courses and for nurses and some other groups post-basic education. Nursing diplomas were introduced and the process was called Project 2000. The emphasis would be as much on the theoretical base and students would be based in higher education with clinical placements, rather than working on the wards with periods in the classroom.

These changes were and have remained controversial. What is less well remembered is that employers were meant to adapt to new recruits whose skill base on qualification would differ from those who qualified under the existing system.

There was little experience of contracting for education within the NHS and little national advice or consistency. The process was rapid in some areas, slow in others. Competitive tendering, when rigorously applied, did affect badly relationships between the NHS and higher education, which in some cases took many years to get over.

The eleventh working paper, which was unnumbered, dealt with medicine and dentistry. It, too, revolutionized the way education and training was funded and managed in these disciplines. The postgraduate medical deans who since the 1960s had educational and pastoral responsibility for postgraduate medical education were given considerable financial and managerial power. They were given budgets covering part of the basic salary of all full-time hospital trainees (and the full basic salary of part-time trainees); the costs of running the local postgraduate medical centres and libraries in hospitals; the cost of study leave and removal costs as well as that of their own management needs including the networks of clinical tutors. There was a rapid expansion of deaneries to cover the educational networks with associate deans, speciality training committee chairmen and medical personnel and financial expertise being added to deaneries. In hospital practice, there was clear commitment to fund the direct costs of postgraduate education, but not the indirect costs such as consultant time. Whereas postgraduate education was funded through the Deans, that of the continuing education of consultant and non-consultant career-grade staff was left with the hospitals. This was the start of the internal market and trusts were instructed to build the cost of chief medical examiners (CMEs) into their contracts. Few did so formally!

In general practice, the working paper brought the then regional advisers in general practice and their networks of course organizers, who looked after vocational training, and GP tutors who, in contrast to the hospital sector, had responsibility for the career grades, into the structure of the overall postgraduate deanery. The regional advisers' networks were further supported by the overall flow of funds into the deaneries. In primary care, the responsibility for training other professionals and, indeed, all other staff lay with health authorities or the practices themselves. Working paper 10 was entirely focused on hospital and community service staff and formally excluded general medical services. Informally, some regional health authorities did begin to support the training of practice nurses, but this was patchy.

The other main national funding stream was the Service Increment for Teaching (SIFT), which had been introduced in 1977 to support the excess costs incurred by the teaching hospitals in providing clinical places for medical students. In 1991, no SIFT went to general practice for teaching medical students and the numbers taught in this setting were low. SIFT and its successor, SIFTR, which contained an added element for research (the 'R' component), is covered in more detail below.

Current organization and funding

The systems described above led in 1996 to the establishment of three national education and training levies for England. These were SIFT covering medical and dental students (the Medical and Dental Education Levy— MADEL), Postgraduate Medical and Dental Education (or PGMDE), and, finally, the Non-medical Education and Training (or NMET) levy covering a range of clinical professionals other than doctors and dentists, notably nurses, midwives, therapists, clinical psychologists, and scientists. Other groups such as speech and language therapists and medical laboratory scientists have been added to NMET since its inception. To these three levies must be added what is often described as the fourth levy, namely funds used by health-care providers from their service income to provide training from their employees ranging from cleaners to consultants and funds from health authorities and primary care organizations for the same purpose.

As the name suggests, the education and training levies are levied from Health Authority allocations. Each Health Authority knows how much has been levied. Before the levies were introduced, the funding for NHS education and training was top sliced centrally before any service allocations were made. These national levies are compulsory and there is no guarantee that any locality will get back what was levied from it.

SIFT

SIFT was introduced in 1977 to support the additional costs incurred by teaching hospitals in teaching medical students. A research component was later added to cover research infrastructure costs creating SIFTR. In 1996, following reviews of both research funding and of SIFT, the two were separated and 25% of the total SIFTR was put into a separate R&D levy. This is not discussed further here. The SIFT review, 'SIFT into the Future', confirmed the function of SIFT as meeting 'the demonstrated excess costs of teaching medical students on clinical placements'. SIFT was divided into a variable portion (20%) termed placements, which was to follow the student and a relatively fixed portion (80%) termed facilities, which was meant to represent the embedded infrastructure costs of teaching. Where appropriate, SIFT could be applied to any organization that taught medical students, including general practice. Furthermore, payments already being made from the NHS to general practice, such as tasked funding and small GP payments, were consolidated into SIFT as was the small sessional payment of £12 that had been agreed for GPs who taught students. The full amount for each full-time equivalent student placement is now just over £9000 in London, a little less elsewhere. Over the succeeding years, the proportion of placements SIFT going into general practice teaching has risen significantly in London, from an average of under 3% in 1996 to 10% in 2000/01. Some practices also receive facilities funding though as yet this is patchy across the country. Increasing facilities SIFT for general practice teaching is difficult because the percentage drop in teaching hospital numbers makes little difference to their embedded infrastructure costs.

The national budget holder for SIFT has been the Chief Medical Officer, with the regional directors holding the regional budget. This has been delegated increasingly to regional directors of education and training or in some cases to regional finance directorates. From 2001, SIFT will form one part of the Multi-professional Education and Training (MPET) levy held nationally by the NHS Executive Director of Human Resources.

MADEL

This levy covers PGMDE. It has six main headings: the funding of training posts, of local PGMDE facilities, such as postgraduate centres and libraries and study leave, public health doctors' training, the costs of the deans managerial infrastructure, the educational networks, and, most recently, the costs of GP registrars and their training. This was moved into MADEL from the General Medical Services (GMS) budget recently. Within the overall budget lies the cost of the directors of postgraduate GP education and their networks of course organizers, GP tutors, and trainers and that part of the dental deans' allocation that comes through MADEL. The postgraduate deans, dental deans and GP directors manage the process of PGMDE, ensuring that standards are met, supporting and following individual trainees to ensure they reach the accreditation standards, inspecting and approving Pre-registration House Officer (PRHO) and Senior House Officer (SHO) posts and working with the medical royal colleges on GP training and on higher specialist training. At national level there are UK-wide committees where medical and dental deans and the GP directors, respectively, meet the health departments to discuss the development and implementation of policy.

The transfer of funding for GP registrars from GMS to MADEL puts more control of GP training in the hands of the GP directors, while making them work more closely with health authorities. The SHO posts used in vocational training still lie uncomfortably between the hospital and general practice and medical workforce planning for general practice still revolves around the medical practitioner committees. The forthcoming review of primary care workforce planning, which will complete the work started by 'A Health Service of all the Talents'[2], will hopefully address this issue. The current intention is to move MADEL into the MPET levy in 2002.

NMET

NMET is the most complex and far ranging of the levies, relying as so much of it does on legally binding contracts between the NHS and higher education for the provision of both pre- and post-qualification education provision. With the introduction of the levy came the development of the education and training consortia. These were local groups of employers of NHS-trained staff together with the commissioners of health-care services, the health authorities. The intention was to include not only NHS employers, but also social services and the independent and voluntary sector. The consortium's prime role was to take over from the disbanded regional health authorities the contracts with higher education. The consortia were not legal entities and so one of the members acted as lead body, employing consortium staff and paying the bills. The lead body was linked to the other NHS members through a series of collateral agreements and called down NMET funds from one of the member health authorities. This apparently clumsy system has in fact worked remarkably well. Most of the NMET expenditure is on the education contracts and on the student bursaries given to students on these courses.

A major problem for primary care when NMET was first introduced was that it was directed at Hospital and

Community Services and did not cover General Medical Services. However, in 1998, NMET was restructured into core and specialist and development components. The core included all pre-qualification education for nurses and other groups. Contracts and bursaries within core NMET account for 80–85% of total NMET expenditure. The specialist component covered the post-qualification contracts that had traditionally consisted of English National Board approved nursing courses. The development component covered everything else, but allowed for greater flexibility in the use of NMET, for example, in primary care. The education and training consortia were created at a time when the new primary care structure of primary care groups and trusts had not been created. Their tradition was rooted in the hospital and community sector. It is therefore very important that primary care education leaders take advantage of the new workforce development confederations described below to raise the profile and needs of education and training for all primary care staff and learn to use these broader systems effectively.

Complexities arose with the three levies because each had its own rules, some of which contradict each other. An example of this is that SIFT pays for clinical placements, whereas NMET does not. Finding sufficient suitable clinical placements in primary care for nurses and therapists is consequently a problem but also a necessity to train the workforce for the future. Some of the complexity is understandable when viewed from a historical perspective—understandable, but not acceptable. The creation of the MPET levy, albeit with the three existing funding streams, is the first small step to unifying and simplifying the whole funding system.

Current and future changes

This is a time of change in primary care education with new initiatives from the Department of Health and the Department for Education and Skills (formerly the Department of Education and Employment) altering the content, method of delivery, and philosophy around education, training, and personal development. There is now clear recognition and backing for lifelong learning as essential to personal fulfilment and personal and national prosperity.

Some of the new education and training organizations are in their infancy and only came into existence in April 2001. These organizations will support the continuum of learning from pre-registration, undergraduate or basic training to continuing personal development for all primary care staff, as well as hospital and community staff. Some of their roles and structures are evolving and will change over the next few years. Nevertheless, there are a large number of organizations who can and should be used by individuals working in primary care or be used by primary care organizations to support all those working in them.

Workforce development confederations

Workforce development confederations have taken over and will expand the functions of education and training consortia from the spring of 2001. They have three broad areas of work including the education and training of all health-care staff whether they are working in the NHS, social services, voluntary, or private sectors. They will be responsible for the workforce planning of all staff working in all sectors of health care. They will also take over supra-employer human resource management issues where it is

appropriate to do so, for example, recruitment and retention initiatives, including overseas recruitment. Finally,
they will play a role in the quality assurance of all non-
medical education and training working with the appropriate national bodies.

The whole of England is covered by 24 workforce development confederations. They will be hosted by a health
authority and be managed by a top team of a chief executive, a finance director and a head of workforce development. Initially they will manage the resources for the
development of all non-medical staff but from April 2002
they will also manage resources for undergraduate and
postgraduate medical staff. They will gradually develop
expertise about all local education and training organizations inside and outside the NHS and therefore be an
important source of advice for individuals and organizations wishing to access education, training, or personal
development, or the resources to support them. Not only
will they commission, organize, and develop expertise in
education and training, but as a confederation of local
health-care organizations they will also provide the placements for the training of staff. In medical education, as
they take over funding, they will gradually work closer
with postgraduate medical deaneries and the medical
schools. The Postgraduate Dean will be a full member of
the confederation boards. Primary care trusts will be full
members of confederations.

Postgraduate medical deaneries

Under the leadership of the Postgraduate Dean, the postgraduate medical deaneries continue to be responsible for
the education and training and quality assurance of the

training of postgraduate doctors. The deanery senior team continue to be supported by networks of educators and committees and a deanery office. The Director of Postgraduate General Practice Education continues to have responsibility for the vocation training for general practice and continuing professional development of general practitioners. They are increasingly becoming involved in the education of other doctors working in primary care and supporting doctors whose performance is causing concern or found to be lacking by the NHS or the GMC. The Directors of Postgraduate GP Education also continue to be supported by a network of course organizers who manage the vocational training of doctors for general practice and GP tutors who manage the provision and quality assurance of continuing professional development for GPs. Both groups of medical educationist are increasingly working with other professionals whose role is to manage or provide education and training for other professional staff within primary care. These nurse or support staff facilitators are currently resourced either by funding from health authorities plus in the future from workforce development confederations.

Whilst the Postgraduate Dean has overall responsibility for the management of postgraduate medical education and its quality assurance, the Director of Postgraduate GP Education is directly responsible for the quality of vocational training and continuing professional development for general practitioners. The Specialist Training Authority or the Joint Committee for Postgraduate Training in General Practice (see later) externally validates the quality of medical education.

Over time, the workforce development confederations and postgraduate deaneries are likely to work increasingly together, particularly in their office function, in workforce planning and allocation of funding. However, the

Postgraduate Dean and the Director of Postgraduate GP Education will remain accountable for the management of postgraduate medical education and its quality.

NHS Trust education centres

The NHS is a major provider of in-house education and training for all staff groups. NHS trusts are increasingly identifying a senior manager at board level to take charge of the overall management of education training and personal development within their organization. Working to this individual are expanding groups of staff members who are responsible for lifelong learning for all staff groups, the provision of student placements and their quality for undergraduate students or postgraduate professional staff trainees. Most trusts have a staff member whose responsibility is the continuing development of support staff. Much educational activity continues to be provided within education centres and supported by library services. However, with the development of information technology and the ability to access learning online, all staff groups are increasingly able to access learning in other ways. Information technology offers an opportunity for primary care staff to increase their ability to access work-based learning (see University for Industry/Learn Direct later).

Primary care groups/primary care trusts

Primary care groups or trusts are or will increasingly be taking responsibility for the strategic management of education and training and personal development for all staff groups. They will need to ensure that primary care staff have access to learning at least equal to that of staff working in hospital trusts. IT-based learning, plus the development of a similar infrastructure to hospital trusts, will help them fulfil this obligation. All organizations within primary care will also be playing their part in the development of future staff by the provision of placements for both undergraduate students and postgraduate trainees. Primary care groups and trusts should play a full part in workforce development confederations and can call on both the confederations and the postgraduate medical deaneries to offer the expert support to develop learning opportunities for staff.

In areas of social and health deprivation, whose recruitment to good practice can be poor, Teaching Primary Care Trusts are being established that will provide an academic base to attract recruits and develop primary care.

Department of Health

The Department of Health (DH) has a role in advising ministers on policy around lifelong learning, education, and training and also has responsibilities in the national overall organization and regulation of education and training.

Currently, each region has appointed a Director of Workforce Development, whose responsibilities include education and training and workforce planning. Regional offices and the Director of Workforce Development's primary function is to develop confederations and deaneries to ensure that they carry out their functions within overall government policy and distribute resources to offer an equality of access to all staff wherever they work within the NHS.

Regional offices also compliment educational developments carried out at a local level by funding leading-edge initiatives that take developments further than that currently available locally. Regional offices will continue with these functions until they cease to exist in 2003.

Within the DH, education and training and lifelong learning are a responsibility of the Education and Training Division. This division will ultimately take responsibility for the education and training of all professional staff working in health care.

Quality assurance of undergraduate/ pre-registration education

The quality assurance of undergraduate or pre-registration education training is a partnership between the Quality Assurance Agency (QAA), the appropriate statutory body, the NHS and the DH. The QAA's primary function is to ensure that the courses are of such a standard that they can be given an academic award. The professional or statutory bodies' primary responsibility is to ensure those courses lead an individual to be fit to practise. The DH and NHS's contribution is to ensure that courses make an individual fit to practise within particular roles in the NHS or other health-care providing organizations (fit for purpose); increasingly the three arms of quality assurance are working together to streamline and coordinate their quality assurance mechanisms to ensure fitness for award, practise and purpose.

In postgraduate or post-registration education and training, the current three bodies ensuring fitness to practise are the Joint Committee for Postgraduate Training for General Practice (JCPTGP), the Specialist Training Authority (STA) and the English National Board (ENB). All these bodies are due to be replaced by new mechanisms within the next few years. JCPTGP and the STA are due to evolve into a Medical Standards Board (MESB) who, supported by the medical royal colleges, will quality assure and externally validate programmes of learning for postgraduate doctors.

When there are problems in the future with the education and training of professional staff, there will therefore be three layers to which an individual or organization can turn for resolution of these problems: first, the providers of education and training; second, those that either commission or manage that training (the workforce development confederations and postgraduate deaneries); and ultimately, the national statutory bodies or the DH.

University and higher education sector

Virtually all clinical professional education is now carried in the higher education sector. The numbers in training are going through a rapid expansion. It is probably true to say that training of staff is still over-dominated by the hospital sector and primary care has a role to play in balancing the opportunities for training placements outside hospitals. The opportunity also exists to influence the content of undergraduate and pre-registration curriculum by playing a full part in the workforce development confederations. There is also an increasing exploitation of opportunities for different health professional groups to learn together with the hope that greater understanding will improve the effectiveness of joint working.

The trend continues for increasing numbers of medical

students to spend a higher proportion of their training in primary care settings. All medical schools have a department of primary care or general practice. These departments not only manage the undergraduate medical training that occurs in primary care, but are also increasing the capacity through research networks to generate research in the primary care setting and disseminate research skills. Most primary care departments work in partnership with the postgraduate training practices, practices taking undergraduate students and practices carrying out primary care research. Undergraduate medical education is primarily funded by the Higher Education Funding Council, although the opportunity costs of placements in the NHS will continue to be funded by the SIFT levy, and in the future, the MPET levy.

Further education

Local further education colleges often provide courses that are appropriate for support staff in primary care and training in specific skills, especially IT. Support staff are able to access funding for individual learning via individual learning accounts. Currently such accounts give access to £150 from the Department for Education and Skills. The NHS is topping up this individual learning account by a further £150 and gradually developing the infrastructure to support the development of support staff via individual learning accounts or funded NVQs (national vocational qualifications). Advice for accessing these resources is via the workforce development confederations or NHS local education centres.

Other relevant organizations

The Department for Education and Skills has set up, throughout England, learning and skills councils (who have taken over from the training and enterprise councils) whose responsibility is the management and distribution of resources for education and training of a wide variety of staff from all sectors of industry including staff working in the NHS and primary care. Learning and skill councils have representatives from all local employers and this can include the NHS. They will increasingly become an important source of resource and support for education training and lifelong learning and now have control of local further education funding.

In the policy document 'The Learning Age'[3], the DFEE announced amongst other things the formation of the University for Industry/Learn Direct. Learn Direct offers access to learning, frequently using IT, via a network of local centres and networks of centres associated with sectors of industry, including the NHS. Learning opportunities are available in basic skills including IT, customer care, etc., and would be highly appropriate for support staff in primary care. The Learn Direct NHS centres are currently being piloted in each region and offer access to this learning to staff in the NHS hospitals, but could offer learning to staff in surrounding primary care settings. Often these centres are integrated in other learning facilities for staff within NHS trusts.

Conclusions

There are a wide variety of organizations which need to be understood by those hoping to support primary care staff in their initial undergraduate, pre-registration education and training or lifelong learning. Expert advice can be obtained from workforce development confederations, postgraduate medical deaneries or NHS education centres and this advice will be gradually developed within primary care trusts. All NHS organizations are building up infrastructure to manage the NHS contributions to the training of future staff and the lifelong learning of current staff; this will apply equally to primary care trusts (who should be key representatives for primary care in workforce development confederations) as well as hospital trusts.

References

1. Department of Health. *Working for Patients*. London: HMSO, 1989.
2. Department of Health. *A health service of all the talents: developing the NHS workforce: consultation document on the review of workforce planning*. Leeds: Department of Health, 2000.
3. Department for Education and Employment. *The Learning Age: a renaissance for a new Britain. Presented to Parliament by the Secretary of State for Education and Employment by Command of her Majesty*. London: The Stationery Office, 1998.

2 Education and training for primary care organizations

NEIL JOHNSON

Background and principles

There are two major challenges in relation to education and training to the primary care organizations (PCOs) that are developing in the United Kingdom. The first centres on the responsibility of these organizations for the development of individuals to serve in the current and future health service workforce. The second centres on the need for organizations to maintain the development of the organization. This chapter examines these two issues.

In the United Kingdom, considerable emphasis has been placed on rooting training for the health professions within the service itself. The rationale for this is that, whilst some knowledge, skills, and attitudes can be developed in a classroom setting, the complexity of patient care and the individuality of patients demand that those training for these professions must learn to apply their learning to the care of individual patients. To do this they need to observe experienced practitioners and to practise the application of their learning. As a consequence virtually all of the post-basic training, and increasingly much of the basic training, for the health-care professions takes place in a service setting. Whilst this places a considerable responsibility on the service to provide effective training, it also offers those who provide the service very significant opportunities to influence the health-care workforce of the future. For these reasons, as PCOs take on an increasing role in driving the provision of an effective health-care service, it is crucial that they also ensure that adequate provision is made for the education and training of both the current and the future workforce. PCOs have two main responsibilities. First the PCO will need to provide placements for the training of practitioners preparing for independent practice. Second, in its role as an employer, the PCO will need to support the continuing development of those who work within the organization. This chapter considers these two areas in detail. PCOs will also need to take account of education and training needs in their commissioning of secondary and tertiary care, but this is not considered in detail in this chapter.

PCOs must also consider how the development of the organization as a whole will be maintained. Some might argue that, because organizations are essentially made up of many individuals, if those individuals are allowed to develop, the organization itself will flourish. However, many would argue that without a clear plan for how the organization itself is to move forward, the uncoordinated development of the many will gradually reduce the organization itself to chaos. If this argument is accepted, there is a clear responsibility on those who lead the organization to ensure that the development of the organization is a high priority. This issue, in particular the need for leadership, is considered in more detail in the final section of this chapter.

Developing individuals

Training placements

The number

A combination of the need to expand the health-care workforce and a recognition that experience in primary care is important for many of those entering the health-care professions has resulted in a marked increase in the demand for suitable training placements in PCOs. As shown in Table 2.1, placements are now needed for basic

Table 2.1 Examples of training placements required in primary care

Stage of training	Examples
Basic	Pharmacy
	Health-care assistant
	Physiotherapy
	Occupational therapy
	Dietetics
	Social work
	Nursing
	Medical
Post-basic	Psychology
	Health-care management
	Medical
	Pre-registration House Officer
	Specialist Registrar in Psychiatry
Specialty	Health visiting
	Community nursing
	Practice Nurse
	GP Registrar
	Specialist Registrar in Community Paediatrics

training, for post-basic experience for a wide range of individuals, as well as for specialty training for those planning to pursue a career in a primary care setting. Frequently a number of placements are drawn together to form a coherent 'training programme'.

PCOs need to consider within their plans for the development of their organization how this demand can be met, both now and in the future. For example, whilst the number of practices approved for GP Registrar training nationally is just sufficient to meet the current demand for GP Registrar training, it is not sufficient to meet the likely needs over the next 3 years;[1] most nursing and medical schools are currently expanding their capacity, but few if any are able to provide the number of placements needed in primary care. Consequently, PCOs need to be considering, in conjunction with those responsible for the provision of training (typically the higher education institutes and the workforce confederations on behalf of the NHS regional offices), exactly what the local level of demand is now and is likely to be and how any shortfall can be met. These plans can then form part of the PCO Development Plan.

Because it can take some time (typically 2 years) to prepare an organization and the individuals within it, the need to plan well ahead cannot be over-emphasized; this is just as important when planning the succession in organizations already approved for training as it is when organizations are first contemplating becoming involved in training.

Ensuring quality

However, the issue of capacity is not simply one of the number of placement opportunities. It is vital that these placements offer training of adequate quality. The standards for the quality of training, and the procedures for checking that those standards are being met, are set by a number of bodies—typically those commissioning the training placements (e.g. the workforce confederations, postgraduate deaneries, and higher education institutes). The standards and procedures will often be strongly influenced by national professional bodies (e.g. the colleges and councils).

The quality of placements is usually considered in two ways. First, are the facilities adequate to allow effective training to take place? Second, is the process of training effective? The first of these is about structure and is likely to prove relatively easy to define and measure; however, whilst inadequate facilities may well hamper training, good facilities will not necessarily result in good training. The second is about process (and ultimately outcome), and is considerably more challenging to define, and often difficult to measure; nevertheless, whilst inadequate processes will also hinder training, good processes are more likely to have a positive effect on training. The risk is that, whilst processes are more important, effort may be focused on structure because it is easier to measure.

Table 2.2 lists some examples of the structural elements that are important to good training.

Although there is great debate about exactly what the elements of good training are, a number of examples are:[2]

- a planned individual curriculum, drawing on published curricula and balanced with the educational needs of the individual;
- a variety of teaching methods chosen to reflect the learning style of the learner, the subject matter, and the stage of learning;
- curriculum and teaching methods negotiated between the teacher and the learner;
- regular review of educational progress ('educational appraisal') that considers progress in relation to the

Table 2.2 Examples of good training structures.

Accommodation	Adequate room in which to see patients
	Acceptable residential accommodation
Equipment	Appropriate clinical equipment
Patient records	Access to full, legible, and organized records
Education	Access to facilities to support learning – library, IT, journals
	Regular protected time for personal learning
	Regular protected time for educational supervision
	Learning records maintained
Personnel	Suitable models of team care being demonstrated

curriculum planned and results in plans for learning and review of the curriculum;
• adequate recording of these processes;
• effective relationships achieved and maintained between supervisor and learners;
• models of practice that the learner observes consistent with the teaching;
• regular evaluation of the effectiveness of the teaching.

To support the development of effective training environments, PCOs will need to be able to support development in both structure and process. This support can take a number of forms:

• The PCO could provide financial and personnel resources to address structural shortcomings (e.g. by summarizing medical and nursing records to an appropriate standard).
• The PCO can encourage and resource suitable individuals to undertake the initial and continuing training necessary to become an effective educational supervisor.

• The PCO can link with the appropriate bodies to obtain information about the standards that are required for training and to arrange the application for approval.

Standards are set by a number of bodies,[3,4] but information about them can usually be accessed through the workforce confederations, postgraduate deaneries, the professional bodies (such as royal colleges), or the higher education institutes.

Continuing professional development (CPD)

All organizations in the NHS are now required to ensure that the staff for whom they are responsible are involved in a suitable process to ensure that they maintain and update the skills necessary for their work.[5] The implication is that this will apply not only to all those who are actually employed by the organization, but also to those who find themselves in a more indirect relationship with these organizations—in particular general practitioners and the staff employed by them.

This is to be done through a process based on 'personal development plans' (PDPs), in which individuals identify what they need to learn, plan how they are going to learn, implement their plans, and then follow them up. This approach is strongly supported both by theories on how adults learn best[6] and by evidence that suggests that learning for those working in health care is most productive when it is planned effectively.[7]

At the same time, the bodies responsible for setting and policing the standards of clinical practitioners are increasingly moving to the position of requiring those who are registered with them to produce, on a regular basis, evidence that they are still performing at an acceptable level.

These processes, known variously as revalidation, re-certi-fication or re-accreditation, always require some evidence that the individual practitioner is maintaining their knowledge and skills through some form of continuing professional development. This requirement has put even greater emphasis on the need for effective CPD for all.

A staged approach to development planning—the stages

There are four major stages that underpin effective CPD.

Step 1—identifying needs

The identification of what needs to be learned can be done in many ways.[8] Some of the most common are:

- appraisal and performance review
- audit
- critical incident surveys
- diaries
- gap analysis
- knowledgeable patients
- mentoring
- mistakes
- objective tests
- observation
- organizational business plan
- patient satisfaction surveys
- peer review
- re-certification/re-validation activities
- research
- teaching.

The great temptation when identifying needs is to con-sider only those aspects of our work with which we already feel comfortable, and to ignore those areas that regularly cause us difficulty. If we do this, we gradually develop our knowledge and skills in some areas to very high degrees, but at the cost of our abilities in those areas that we perhaps like less. It is therefore essential that when needs are identified, the process is *comprehensive* (i.e. it covers all aspects of our work) and *searching* (i.e. it covers each aspect in sufficient depth).

To achieve these two aims, two approaches are of particular help. The first is to use an accepted description of the work done by the individual as a basis for the review of needs; the use of a job description or something similar can be very helpful. Examples include the job descriptions used at the appointment of nursing or administrative staff, and the booklet *Good Medical Practice for General Practitioners.*[9] The second is to use a formal appraisal process in which one individual (the appraiser) helps the other (the appraisee) to look at their work; the appraiser can help to ensure that the process is comprehensive and searching. One of the most helpful definitions of the purpose of appraisal has been provided by the General Medical Council.[10] It is essential, if appraisal is to work, that suitable appraisers are identified and that all have appropriate training in appraisal methods; the opportunity for this training is something that all primary care organizations must be prepared to provide.

Step 2—drawing up a plan
One of the main outcomes of needs assesssment or appraisal should be a written record of the educational needs that have been identified. This then needs to be converted into a plan that the individual can use.

To do this, consideration should now be given as to the best way of addressing these needs. When doing this it is important to recognize that we each learn in different ways, and that different subjects may lend themselves to different methods for learning. For example, some people learn by trying a new technique whilst others learn by reading about it.[11] To help an individual decide the way in which they are most likely to learn it is worth looking at a variety of ways in which they might learn,[8] and also looking at the ways that they have found most successful when they have tried to learn in the past. The following are some examples of ways in which learning might take place:[8]

- academic activities, e.g. teaching
- attachments and secondments
- case review
- conferences/meetings
- distance learning
- IT methods
- library work
- opportunistic learning
- reflective learning
- team-based activities
- videotape review of performance
- visits.

Similarly some subjects lend themselves to some methods much more readily than to others—for example, it is usually best to help people to learn how to use a new computer program by giving them an opportunity to try the program for themselves; similarly aspects of team-working are often best learned by giving people the opportunity to work in teams and then reflect on what they have learned and how.

This means that the plan should contain two major components: the subject matter (*content*) and the way in which it is to be learned (*method*).

Step 3—implementing the plan

Once plans have been drawn up, each individual needs to ensure that the plans are implemented. Although this is the responsibility of the individual, some support may be needed. Individuals may need help to find suitable learning activities; they may need to be encouraged to try a new way of learning; they may need to discuss their learning. It is important that primary care organizations make sure that sufficient support is available. Whilst they should consider employing personnel and setting up resource centres to do this, support is likely to be available through the local higher education institutions, the workforce confederations, and the local postgraduate deaneries.

Step 4—following up and recording the learning
Follow-up is important for a number of reasons. First, there is evidence that learning is more likely to be incorporated into everyday practice if the learner takes the time to reflect on how the learning should affect their practice and reflects later on whether it has changed their practice.[8] Second, sharing the learning with others offers the chance for learning to spread beyond the individual learner. Third, records of learning are increasingly becoming a requirement for professional bodies.

It is also important to recognize that not all learning can be planned in advance. Unplanned, or part-planned, learning is likely to be far more effective if the individual puts time aside to reflect on the implications of that learning and also keeps a record of that learning.

Personal development plans and practice/personal development plans

In the section above, consideration has been given solely to individual learners. But few people working in primary care organizations now work alone—the vast majority work in practices that in turn make up the main elements of the primary care organizations, and these organizations will also have plans for their development.

The crucial message is that the principles to be used in development planning for an organization are exactly the same as those used for personal development plans. Needs must be identified, plans drawn up and implemented, and follow-up instituted.

The principal challenge for organizations in drawing up plans is to achieve balance. The aspirations of individuals must be balanced by the needs of other individuals and by the needs of the local community (for example, as defined in the local 'Health Improvement Plan') and the NHS as a whole. To achieve such a balance two approaches are available. The first is for the organization to identify the needs of the population it serves and to draw up its strategy to meet those needs; this is then cascaded down to the individual level. A significant part of each individual's plan is then focused on meeting the objectives of the organization. The second is for the organization to draw together the plans produced by each individual to form the organizational plan. In general, the first approach is preferable because it enables the broadest view of the needs of the population to be taken, and can be used to ensure that all the aspects are addressed. The most significant disadvantage of this approach is that individuals may be left feeling that their personal needs are not being addressed, may then feel undervalued by the organization, and in turn may disengage themselves from the process. For these reasons, the approach chosen will be strongly influenced by the maturity of the organization—the new organization with relatively unsophisticated means for identifying population needs and a desire to ensure that all individuals are engaged may well start with the second approach. If this approach is taken, it is important that ways of resolving potentially competing individual priorities have been agreed before plans are brought together; this will enable individuals to test their personal priorities against this agreed process.

Having drawn up plans, the next major challenge for the organization is to ensure an integrated approach to implementation. Integration should be considered in two ways. First, learning should become an integral part of the normal work of all those involved in the organization; it should not be added on to the usual weekly work. Second, where possible, the learning of different individuals should be integrated—whenever a subject lends itself to joint learning this should be used.

Those responsible for leading the development of the organization and the individuals within it will want to review on a regular basis the degree to which their approach is working. Short-term measures of success will include the extent to which planning is taking place, and the extent to which the records demonstrate that the learning within the organization is balanced and integrated. In the longer term, an assessment will need to be made of the extent to which the population needs identified are being effectively addressed by the organization.

Resources

It is clear that development, both of individuals and of the organization, places a significant responsibility on primary care organizations. The situation is further complicated by the history of rather different approaches to continuing development that have been taken by the individuals and practices that find themselves in these organizations. It is therefore essential that personnel with the necessary skills are available to support this process.

A number of skills will be vital to the successful introduction of both individual CPD and organizational development. In particular, it will be important that the following skills are available:

- personal appraisal (see also Chapters 6 and 7)
- population needs assessment
- understanding of how individuals develop

- understanding of how organizations develop
- facilitation (personal and group)
- evaluation of learning
- leadership.

It is not crucial for all these skills to be invested in a single individual, nor is it essential that all these skills are available from within the organization itself. It is highly likely that the skills will be shared amongst a number of people and that some of these individuals will be employed by other organizations; through partnership with these organizations it should be possible to ensure that all these skills are available throughout the organization. Nevertheless, of this list the one set of skills that really do need to be available from within the organization are those relating to the provision of leadership—without leadership it will be extremely difficult to introduce and maintain the continuing development of individuals and the organization. This is considered in more detail in the final section of this chapter.

In addition to these skills, a number of publications are now available which can be used to support CPD.[12,13]

Developing the organization

Just as individuals need to develop, so too do the organizations within which they work. But whilst the principles of development are common to individuals and to organizations, there is one major difference. If an organization is to move forwards, it needs to have a clear purpose and a set of goals and principles that are shared and accepted by those who work within it—it needs to function as a community and not simply as a conglomeration of individuals.[14] In order to maintain its purpose and principles and ensure movement towards its intended goals, the organization needs effective leadership.

Goals, purpose, and principles

Successful organizations are frequently identified as having 'vision'. Although it is not always clear what is meant by this term, Bennis and Nanus[15] have defined vision as the integration of goals (the direction in which the organization is moving) that are founded on a core purpose (what the organization is there to do) and a set of core principles (the set of guiding rules by which the organization abides). The organization is encouraged to move forward (towards its goals) whilst remaining rooted in firm foundations (its purpose and principles). The term 'strategy' is also used. Strategy is the term usually used when a vision has been converted into a set of specific activities for implementation. Strategy also flows from the same three elements—the organization clarifies what it must continue to do and what it wishes to do to if the core purpose is to be met as fully as possible, the whole being underpinned by a framework of principles. A brief example of a strategy based on these three elements is given in Box 2.1.

It is important to recognize that, particularly within a public service such as the NHS, goals, purpose, and principles are likely to arise both from within the organization and from outside of the organization. For PCOs in the UK, outline goals will frequently be defined by national or regional health initiatives (e.g. the National Service Frameworks); this does not mean that there is no scope for local initiative as it is frequently possible for individual PCOs to shape both the exact goals and the way by which they will be achieved. Similarly, a national framework of

Box 2.1   Example of a strategy incorporating goals, purpose, and principles

Organization

- A Postgraduate Medical Deanery responsible for the training of doctors.

Purpose

- 'The core purpose of this organization is to promote the delivery of high quality patient care through the provision of a medical workforce skilled to provide high quality in all aspects of care'.

Principles

This strategy is underpinned by the following principles:
- keeping patients and their care as the central concern;
- striving for excellence;
- being supportive to individuals and to organizations wherever possible;
- having systems that are fair, equitable, transparent, and efficient;
- working with other organizations wherever appropriate;
- being flexible in approach and response.

Goals for this year

- Developing new training posts in areas highlighted by assessment of patient need
- Introduction of educational programmes to develop particular skills to address the needs of patients – in particular communication skills and change management skills
- Introduction of new quality assurance systems for the training programmes
- Recruiting and training new trainers

purpose and principles has been defined for the NHS;[1] again the PCO can augment these purposes and principles with particular ones for its own working (provided that they do not conflict with those agreed nationally).

Once the final vision and strategy has been agreed, it is important that all those within the organization understand what is planned. It is therefore important to share a strategy document with all who will be involved in the delivery of the strategy. This will enable them to see where their activities fall into the large organizational jigsaw, and will also help them to ensure that their PDPs are consistent with the plans for the organization.

Leadership

Although vision is crucial to successful organizational development, it is not sufficient on its own. It is essential that there is also effective leadership. Part of leadership is the development of vision, but it also involves other activities. In particular:

Leading individuals

- Explaining the current position of the organization and the direction in which it is moving
- Enabling individuals within the organization to share and own the vision
- Supporting future leaders

Leading the organization

- Being trustworthy
- Creating an atmosphere in which improvement is continuously sought
- Managing external relationships (including upwards relationships)

- Maintaining an effective balance between ensuring that the agreed long-term goals are achieved and reacting to short-term situations that arise
- Ensuring that the risks of being innovative and creative are managed appropriately

Because leadership is so central to successful organizations, PCOs should be looking to identify, select, develop and nurture future leaders.

Conclusions

PCOs have a number of responsibilities in relation to education, training, and development—to individuals training for the health service or working within the organization, and to the organization as a whole. They have a major role in supporting the development of training placements by ensuring that they are available in sufficient numbers and that they are of high quality. They need to support the continuing development of individuals through planned, balanced and integrated CPD. This needs to be supplemented by effective organizational development. It requires the organization to identify its core purpose along with its underpinning principles and its goals. To achieve all of this, a number of skills are needed, most significant of which is effective leadership. As PCOs mature, there is a real opportunity for them to develop into institutions in which the opportunity for individuals or the organization as a whole to learn continuously forms one of the core principles underpinning the organization.

References

1. Department of Health. *The NHS Plan*. London: Department of Health, 2000.
2. Havelock P, Hasler J, Flew R *et al*. *Professional Education for General Practice*. Oxford: Oxford University Press, 1995.
3. Royal College of General Practitioners. *Quality Team Development—Standards and Criteria 2000*. London: RCGP, 2000.
4. Joint Committee on Postgraduate Training for General Practice. *Recommendations to Deaneries for the Establishment of Criteria for the Approval and Reapproval of Trainers in General Practice*. London: JCPTGP, 1998.
5. NHS Executive. *Working Together: Securing a Quality Workforce for the NHS*. London: Department of Health, 1998.
6. Schon DA. *The Reflective Practitioner: How Professionals think in Action*. London: Arena, 1991.
7. NHS Centre for Reviews and Dissemination. Getting evidence into practice. *Effective Health Care* 1999; **5**(1).
8. Grant J, Chambers E, Jackson G, eds. *The Good CPD Guide for Medicine*. London: Joint Centre for Education in Medicine, 1999.
9. General Practitioners Committee, Royal College of General Practitioners. *Good Medical Practice for General Practitioners*. London: RCGP, 2000.
10. General Medical Council. Revalidating Doctors: ensuring standards, securing the future. Consultation document. London: GMC, 2000.
11. Kolb DA. The process of experiential learning. In: Thorpe M, Edwards R, Hanson A, eds. *Culture and Processes of Adult Learning*. London: Routledge, 1993.
12. While R, Attwood M, eds. *The Wessex Way: a Framework for Professional Development in Primary Care*. Bath: University of Bath, 1999.
13. Gallen D. *Personal Development Plan: a Practical Aid to getting started on your PDP*. London: Update, 2000.
14. Harvey-Jones J. *Making it Happen: Reflections on Leadership*. London: Harper Collins, 1994.
15. Bennis W, Nanus B. *Leaders*. New York: Harper Perennial, 1985.

3 Interprofessional and multiprofessional education and training in primary care

JONATHAN BURTON,
HELEN PRENTICE, AND TONY WEIGHT

Introduction

For many years, interprofessional education for primary care has been an area for pioneers. Suddenly, it has become an activity that is highly desirable and about to become mainstream. In the stampede to 'go interprofessional', some careful consideration will be needed. We will all need to understand what has worked in the past, how effective learning activities can be stimulated, and what the limitations of interprofessional education are.

Definitions

There is enormous confusion about definitions.[1] For this chapter we are adopting the definitions of interprofessional/multiprofessional which have been put forward by CAIPE. 'Interprofessional education takes place on occasions when two or more professions learn together with the object of cultivating collaborative practice and improving the health and well being of their clients.'[2,3] Multi-professional education, on the other hand, occurs when two or more professions learn together for whatever reason.[2]

The terms interdisciplinary and multidisciplinary education are used in the American literature to describe what is accepted as interprofessional/multiprofessional in the UK literature. There is, however, a practical use, within the Health Service in the UK, of the term multidisciplinary. A multidisciplinary team is a team that has individuals from different professional and non-professional backgrounds, who all exercise different skills for one overall clinical task. For example, a neurocare multidisciplinary team is made up of specialist nurses, occupational therapists, neurologists, physiotherapists, a secretary, and so on. All members of such a team are involved in the care of one patient with a chronic neurological illness.

For this chapter we use the terms interprofessional and multiprofessional and follow the definitions put forward by CAIPE.

The core primary care team and the extended primary care team

Teamwork is central to good care.[4,5] The core primary care team (GP, practice nurse, practice administrative staff) has also to work with a larger group of other health and social care professionals. These are: district nurses, health visitors, social workers/home carers, community mental health teams, learning disability teams, community pharmacists, physiotherapists, hospice teams, and so on, all of these professionals together making up the extended primary care team. Such extended teams are really important for patient care in a number of settings:

- prescribing issues
- child protection issues
- care of the very elderly or very handicapped
- care of patients with terminal illness
- care of patients with serious mental illness/learning disability.

The extended primary care team always works on several sites and has worked historically under several employers: some members never meet together. It is likely that, as primary care organizations (PCOs) develop, most, but not all, of these groups will be brought more closely together in terms of their management and/or employment. Whilst this will make the coordination of services easier, it will not of itself guarantee better delivery of care to patients. Improving patient care will depend on (as it always has) a team approach built on:

- knowledge of the roles of other professionals
- the ability to work with other professionals
- ability of the team to learn together in order to improve care together.

Interprofessional education and training in a changing world

Experiments in interprofessional education and training have occurred in many contexts around the world and an excellent summary of the world picture is available on the CAIPE website.[6] The position of interprofessional education is changing from one that is mainly experimental or additional to uniprofessional education to one that becomes mainstream.

Governments and international agencies seek to modernize health services and to make them appropriate for a developing environment. This is an environment of changing demographics, changing disease patterns, of new technologies and changing expectations. More diseases can be prevented and more diseases can be treated. The pace of change in health services around the world is dictated by these external events.

The professional interests of separate groups are now being more firmly challenged. Important questions are being asked:

- What sort of health professional should deliver what sort of care in the community?
- What sort of education and training will create such professionals?
- And how can health care for individuals and populations be improved?

Interprofessional education and training have become central to these processes of change. Why is this? First, it is because of the need for collaborative practice between the different professions. Teams consisting of individuals from different professions must work efficiently together. Neither of these processes can be achieved without joint learning.

Most challengingly, the rights of each profession to preserve territories of activity in patient care will give way to new ways of working—with, most obviously, nurses taking on roles that have been traditionally performed by doctors and others taking on the roles that have been previously performed by nurses. This process of 'substitution and moving across',[1] which up until now has been largely experimental, will gather pace and interprofessional education and training will play an important part in the process.

A number of influences, both governmental and non-governmental, have in the last 10 years guided changes in:

- the delivery of primary care
- the management of education and training within primary care.

Box 3.1 summarizes the main changes and influences within the UK.

A new, integrated approach to education and training and workforce planning is now planned in the UK. *A Health Service of all the Talents: Developing the NHS Workforce*[7] arose from a highly critical House of Commons Select Committee report on the NHS. This identified the confusion of the three funding streams for education (see Box 3.1), three funding streams which had been established in previous organizational changes but which were seen now to act counter to the aim of providing an efficient service. There is acceptance within *A Health Service of all the Talents* that there is a need for greater clarity about the future requirements for primary care and hence for GP and other primary care staff. The document also clearly indicates the need to plan the Primary Care Workforce in a more informed and integrated way. The staffing crisis in many parts of the NHS has brought the NHS workforce to the top of the agenda for change.

The NHS Plan: a Plan for Investment, a Plan for Reform[8] foresees an integration of Education and Training levies through new organizations to be called confederations: it also foresees a new common core curriculum for all students training for professional roles within the health service.

What will promote interprofessional education and training within primary care?

The six case histories, which follow later in this chapter, are six real-life scenarios involving interprofessional

Box 3.1   Summary of influences in the last decade which have had an impact on primary care, and primary care education and training

Government-led changes

1990 – The New Contract
mid-1990s – Merging of Family Service Health Authorities and Health Authorities
mid-1990s – National levy system funding for education and training

- Levy 1: Medical and Dental Educational Levy (MADEL). Purpose: funding of Vocational Training for GPs and the GP Tutor system. This has not funded the Postgraduate Education Allowance.
- Levy 2: Non-medical Education and Training Levy (NMET). Purpose: included funding of education of primary care professionals other than doctors within its remit. See Case Histories 5 and 6 for some practical details.
- Levy 3: Service Increment for Teaching (SIFT). Purpose: funding of medical education.

1998 – A First-class Service

- Linked the delivery of high-quality care and clinical governance with professional self-regulation and life-long learning.

2000 – A Health Service of all the Talents: developing the NHS Workforce
2000 – The NHS Plan: a Plan for Investment, a Plan for Reform

Other influences

The Pharmaceutical Industry

continued

- Funding from the pharmaceutical industry has been both promotional and non-promotional. The National Training Centre for Asthma was funded by a pharmaceutical company. The role of this industry is well illustrated in the case histories.

The introduction of compulsory or semi-compulsory requirements for on-going learning (PREPs for nurses, PGEA for GPs).

- For all the criticisms of these approaches, they have undoubtedly led to a culture of 'education and life-long learning' where little existed before.

The growth of work-based learning

- Most primary care teams now undertake some in-house education. Read Burton[9] for a definition of work-based learning.
- The evidence-based medicine and guidelines movements. These movements have had a major effect on approaches to learning and practice.

education and training. We, as authors, have been involved in all of them, either because we have participated as clinicians, or because we have management or educational knowledge of them. We do describe the outcomes in each of these initiatives and how each was funded, and we give our opinions as to how much and for what reason each programme has been successful.

Managers of education and training and educationalists themselves need to know what will work best. There are two polarized models of promoting change through education and training, one which is managed from the top and the other which promotes initiative from the grass roots. Similarly, there are two models of funding education and training. The first is where funding is managed from the top downwards. In this model a main funding organization, such as an educational consortium, funds subsidiary organizations, such as colleges or educational boards, which contract to provide stated courses and programmes to 'educate and train' health-care workers. The other model of funding is the bottom-up model. In this model, funding is used to promote local (often work-based) initiatives. In assessing how worthwhile each approach is, it is useful to understand how educational programmes can be evaluated, and, further, to understand which types of programme are likely to achieve the most appropriate changes in patient care. In this chapter, we describe an approach to evaluating education which was first developed by Kirkpatrick[10] (see the next section).

Klein and Dixon[11] have summed up this tension between the managed versus the innovative:

the problem is how to create more 'space' for professionals—to improve their own practices, innovate and learn, communicate their ideas to their colleagues, and, above all, spend more time with patients—while still maintaining the drive to improve efficiency, quality and productivity. The answer may lie in a mixture of selective incentives and selective top-down pressures . . . .

Measuring the effectiveness of interprofessional education

The JET (Joint Evaluation Team) has been reporting for the past 2 years on their extensive enquiry into the effectiveness of interprofessional education. As a framework for measuring effectiveness, they have used their own development of Kirkpatrick's[10] original hierarchy of evaluation. Their framework is summarized in Box 3.2.

Box 3.2   The Joint Evaluation Team's (JET) development of Kirkpatrick's original hierarchy of evaluation[12]

- Level 1: learner's reaction
- Level 2a: modification of knowledge and skills
- Level 2b: acquisition of knowledge and skills
- Level 3: transferring learning to the workplace – behavioural changes
- Level 4a: change in organizational practice
- Level 4b: benefits to patients

Case histories

We have chosen six case histories from our own working knowledge. These have not been chosen to necessarily illustrate the best. Rather they have been chosen to illustrate the variety of ways that health-care staff working in the community have been educated and trained. We gauge the outcome of each of the six initiatives, using the modified Kirkpatrick framework, and give our own opinions as to why success has been achieved. We also describe how the initiatives have been funded.

Case 1

Charting the development of nurses in two general practice settings—1990 to present. The Surgery, Halstead and The Limes Medical Centre, Epping[13]

The New Contract of 1990 gave a major, but somewhat indirect push to the development of the practice nurse role. It emphasized the need to provide anticipatory care: for example, by the setting of targets for immunization and cervical screening, and by the provision of payment for Health Promotion clinics.

Gradually throughout the 1990s the role of practice nurse in both practices has changed.

At The Limes, three practice nurses have trained as Nurse Practitioners (NPs), taking BSc qualifications through the Royal College of Nursing. The Health Authority funded this training. Mentor-ship during this course was provided by GPs in The Limes Medical Centre. The courses were largely theoretical. The practice and local hospitals provided a clinical element of teaching.

At the end of their training, the NPs were able to develop their specialist roles and to undertake ordinary 'surgeries'. Patients were invited to see either a GP or the NP and a patient satisfaction survey was undertaken afterwards. Patients who had seen the NP were highly satisfied —a change at Kirkpatrick level 4b.

One nurse practitioner runs a diabetic clinic with a GP, a chiropodist, and a dietitian. The practice can now look after most newly diagnosed insulin-dependent diabetic patients, by providing a complete community-based service. One nurse practitioner and one GP undertake the whole minor surgery service for the patients in the practice.

The practice has an in-house clinical educational programme that nurses and doctors attend. Some basic funding (for example, for refreshments) is provided by the pharmaceutical industry.

In Halstead, a nurse skilled in diabetes education was originally trained in the 1980s with a Health Authority grant. The hospital-based Diabetes Specialist Nurse provided the training and this was done in the practice. When that practice nurse retired, her successor was trained in exactly the same way. She is able to provide the sort of service to the practice's patients that had traditionally been provided by a hospital specialist nurse.

The practice was involved in a locality action learning project[13] on Parkinson's disease in the community. The local neurology team provided expert input and a pharmaceutical company funded the whole project. As a result of this project and based on a realization of unmet patient needs, a group of local practices decided to appoint a part-time community-based Parkinson's disease (PD) nurse. This is an example of an outcome at Kirkpatrick level 4. This post was funded for the Parkinson's Disease Society and the fund-holding consortium. This nurse was trained on the Parkinson's Disease Society specialist nurse programme. When the local primary care group was set up, the nurse was taken on full time by the PCG as a community-based PD nurse, a post funded by the PCG.

The Halstead practices have a very varied in-house education programme (food and other essentials are funded by pharmaceutical companies but it is otherwise run at zero cost). This is mainly multiprofessional and has four main strands:

- action learning or project-based learning
- seminars with expert input
- annual rolling programmes for audit and diabetes care between five local practices
- individual written projects.

These two stories are stories of practices in which professional roles have developed through innovation. They show how nurses have, with extra training, learned to carry out roles traditionally carried out by doctors, or traditionally performed only in secondary care. The practices continue to provide a learning environment in which, even now, future innovations may have their origin.

Case 2

Cancer care in the community[14]*—funded by locality self-financing education group, a grant from the Health Authority, and a pharmaceutical company (accommodation and food).*

Five primary care teams covering a geographical area of north Essex developed a joint education programme from the mid-1990s. The five practices were members of a fund-holding consortium. The educational programmes were organized by local professionals and at least one programme a year was project based. In the 'cancer care' project, which took place in 1995–96, each of the five practices joined as a team. The teams consisted of at least one of a GP, a district nurse, and a receptionist/practice manager, but also included health visitors, practice nurses, dispensers, community hospital nurses, and community pharmacists. The learning programme was based around the actual history of a real patient with cancer, for whose care the team had been responsible. Outside resources included the local oncologists and facilitators in communication skills. The programme took place over four afternoons but each team held separate meetings to discuss their case. A reflective interview with each team was part of the fourth afternoon and was used to evaluate the course. Four main outcomes were determined. The learners preferred this sort of learning to the traditional didactic fare (after all, they knew where to find clinical information and did not need to be somewhere 'educational' to do that). They valued the chance it had given them to improve teamwork. They valued the chance it had given them to reflect on the emotional needs of users and professionals. And they enjoyed the chance to reflect on the patient's experiences, some of which had been pretty grim.

But had this course actually improved the delivery of care to patients? In 1997 two of the practices, in response to the educational programme, started weekly team meetings to discuss care of patients where the district nurses and health visitors and GPs were jointly involved. This has definitely improved the care of, for example, patients at home with terminal illness. So a project which when first evaluated showed results up to the modified Kirkpatrick level 2b, in the end has possibly led to changes through levels 3 and 4.

Case 3

The use of Implanon—funded by the device manufacturers

The manufacturers of the contraceptive device, Implanon, offered joint training in its use to doctors and nurses from practices. This gave them the knowledge and skill to both fit the device and counsel patients about the advantages and possible side-effects. Changes at modified Kirkpatrick levels 2b and 3 are likely to have occurred, and possibly at level 4, but any evaluation of the programme is at present unknown.

Case 4

Tailor-made training[15]—funded by a one-off grant from the government-funded LIZEI scheme

This involved 10 primary care teams in north London, who wished to improve their care of diabetes or asthma, and a facilitator. The facilitator was also the researcher. Whilst there was a general structure to the programme, which consisted of nine sessions of an hour or two each, the intervention for each team was tailored to their needs, and built on each team's strengths and dispositions. The programme was mostly directed to enhancing the delivery of care by helping participating teams to see how they could improve organization and team work. The learning agenda was developed after discussing the initial audits in each team and after discussing, in a team setting, the impact of diabetes and asthma on patients and the question of whether the team was working as well as it might. From this discussion a programme for change was devised. Actual 'specialist clinical teaching' was not undertaken by the facilitator but could be undertaken elsewhere as part of the course. The programme was evaluated by before and after audits and by interviews, which were undertaken by the facilitator/researcher and a remarkable level of change was shown. A degree of change at modified Kirkpatrick level 4 had been achieved.

Case 5

The North London Education Consortium and its Primary Care Subgroup (PriSM)

The North London Education Consortium covers Barnet, Camden and Islington, and Enfield and Haringey Health Authority Areas. PriSM, which is a subgroup of the consortium, was established in 1997. It is responsible for developing a strategy for primary health-care education and training for all local health professionals falling within the scope of the NMET levy.

Its five main areas of working are:

• integrating workforce planning
• education and training needs assessment and promoting lifelong learning
• commissioning and arranging education and training, linking them to service needs
• interagency working and resource management
• evaluation of education and training provision.

Membership is drawn from the main consortium, health authorities, GP education boards, community trusts, independent contractors, PCG board lay members and PCG board Local Authority members.

PriSM has an executive, which meets four times a year, and a subgroup which meets three times a year. Its budget for 2000–2001 is £150,000. The budget, however, of the main consortium is very much bigger.

In 1999 and 2000 PriSM has funded a conference at The Tavistock Centre. The 2000 conference was on the subject 'Working Models of Supervision and Support in Primary Care'. GPs, practice nurses and community nurses, and managers attended this conference from a primary care background. The course was mainly experiential and participants were able to get a flavour of mentoring, supervision, consultation-based learning, and so on. Feedback was by questionnaire and was positive but only measured participants' reactions to the course—Kirkpatrick level 1.

Case 6

The North London Consortium, a local education group (CREATES) and the Health Improvement Programmes (HImPS) of 2 PCGs

In 1999–2000, two of Enfield and Haringey's PCGs (Enfield North and Enfield South and Southgate) have diabetes as one of their Health Improvement (HImP) areas. Enfield and Haringey's primary care education group (CREATES), which responds to the educational needs of the PCGs, puts on a study afternoon on diabetes. CREATES receives its funding from the Health Authority and from local GPs.

The study afternoon covers new diabetic guidelines, the UKPDS, and the National Audit of Diabetes. Primary care team staff and community staff attend it. The cost of the afternoon is small as the speakers give their time for free and the main cost is the hire of accommodation and the provision of refreshments. A few community nurses attend and CREATES is able to invoice their nurse manager at £20 a head. The nurse manager has in turn received funding from the main North London Consortium in her year's allocation to pay for such courses.

The community nurses attending the course ask for further training in the 'diabetic foot' and another course on this subject is put on by CREATES. The course is mainly taught by a podiatrist who gives his time for free. The cost per head for community nurses attending the course is claimed by CREATES from the nurse managers, who in turn have received funding for courses from the main consortium. CREATES, as explained above, is funded by the local Health Authority and GPs.

CREATES also puts on an annual, short, academically accredited course on diabetes for nurses. The North London Consortium funds this year by year as part of its 'shopping list' of courses from CREATES. For the whole shopping list it gives CREATES a grant of £20,000. PriSM is not involved in these arrangements and the funding comes from the main Consortium.

Evaluations of these programmes show outcomes limited to Kirkpatrick level 1.

Summary of main points from case histories

- Improvement of care to patients is the 'gold standard' when evaluating educational programmes: in many educational programmes, however, outcomes have not been measured beyond Kirkpatrick level 1 (participants' reactions). Evaluations that indicate improvements in patient care are more likely to occur where the learning has been work based.
- Learning provision in the 'health economy' is varied, some of it self-started and some of it more formally organized.

• Sources of funding for education are: statutory, voluntary organizations, professionals themselves, commercial interests.

The future: designing new ways of working

The UK government, through the NHS Plan[8] and through *A Health Service of all the Talents*[7] is proposing enormous changes in working roles. Professionals will have to 'know about' the roles of other professional groups. They will have to be able to 'work with' other professionals, in the context of a team where each member has a clearly defined role. They will have to be able to 'substitute for' roles traditionally played by other professionals, when circumstances suggest that this would be more effective, and to provide flexibility in career routes: 'moving across'.[1] As described in Box 3.1, the NHS Plan envisages a common core curriculum in some aspects of health care for all those training to become health care professionals. CAIPE[2] has long espoused the advantages of collaborative working, and the GMC,[16] amongst many other groups, fosters the concept that interprofessional learning can contribute to 'a mutual understanding of professional systems, cultures and roles'.

Interprofessional education may foster collaborative working, but is it the most appropriate way of learning? Does our population want to be treated by professionals who excel at collaborative working but who have spent less time in preparing for a precisely defined professional role? Wilson and Mires[17] think that interprofessional learning may impede uniprofessional learning. Their research into limited shared learning between medical students and midwifery students has suggested that though the groups had gained in mutual tolerance, effective learning, which would be appropriate for their future professional roles, had been compromised. In summary, our point about collaborative practice is that though it is desirable in itself, it does not ensure, of itself, that care to patients is improved.

In what setting does interprofessional learning lead to the most clear-cut advantages to the service? Unpublished work by the JET project (Hugh Barr, personal communication) involves an assessment of 163 reported evaluations of interprofessional education (95% of them North American). All the educational interventions were of 2+ weeks. Those involving work-based learning were more likely to report changes in services to patients or the organization of services to patients (modified Kirkpatrick levels 4) than those that were institution-based.

So, whilst many of the Government's policies for the future envisage changes in the way that educational institutions deliver pre-registration education, the evidence for the effectiveness of interprofessional education suggests the following:

- Interprofessional education at pre-registration level can increase mutual understanding and respect.
- Interprofessional education at post-registration level is more effective at changing services to patients when it is work-based.
- There is a danger that too great an emphasis on interprofessional education will reduce the quality of the necessary uniprofessional learning.

Summary

NHS policy continues to move in the direction of interprofessional education and training. If 'modernization' of the NHS is about doing things differently, rather than just doing more of the same, then further innovation and changes are bound to occur in the next few years. For the foreseeable future, the current education and training system will continue to operate at undergraduate level on a uniprofessional basis for entry to a health-care profession. It is increasingly likely, however, that some parts of each profession's curriculum will be seen as needing to be taught together and this will become the norm rather than the exception. However, uniprofessional education must not suffer.

Post-registration learning, also described as lifelong learning, will continue to thrive by innovation. It should increasingly be work based and will, when appropriate, be interprofessional.

National and local imperatives (clinical governance, health improvement programmes, and so on) will continue to influence the curriculum and in many cases will favour interprofessional learning. Whether this will lead to a dilution of the uniqueness of each health-care profession remains to be seen, but some blurring at the boundaries of professional practice is already happening and will continue. For experienced professionals working as a team in primary care, the maxim of optimizing the effectiveness of a team approach will be pursued with increasing enthusiasm. Developments around learning together are likely to have as much impact on primary care as on other health-care sectors. There is evidence in favour of work-based learning for achieving the greatest benefits to patients. Funding streams for education and training will be reorganized but the natural history of successful learning within the primary care setting suggests that managed 'one-stream' funding for education and training, whilst important, may not actually have a significant impact on successful work-based learning. And it is work-based learning which seems to be most effective approach to improving services to patients.

Box 3.3   Summary of main points of chapter

- The CAIPE definitions for interprofessional and multi-professional education are used.
- Interprofessional education and training are part of an international movement, aimed at improving collaboration between the professions and within teams, and to make the delivery of care to patients and populations both appropriate and effective.
- The JET team's evaluation framework, based on Kirkpatrick, is a good way of assessing the effectiveness of educational interventions.
- Interprofessional education and training are central to the plan to 'modernize' the NHS: unifying the different ways of funding education and training within the NHS is one strand of this strategy.
- In pre-registration education and training, interprofessional learning leads to better mutual understanding between the different professional groups. It may, however, harm uniprofessional learning.
- For established health professionals, working in teams, work-based learning is more likely to lead to improvements in patient care than institution-based learning.
- The NHS authorities should seek to encourage work-based learning.

Further reading and information

- CAIPE Bulletin is a must (access the organization through www.caipe.org.uk).

- The Learning Workplace (access the organization and its journal through the website www.tlw.org.uk).

References

1. Finch J. Interprofessional education and teamworking: a view from the education providers. *British Medical Journal* 2000; **321**: 1138–40.
2. CAIPE. Interprofessional education—a definition. *CAIPE Bulletin* 1997; **13**: 19.
3. Zwarenstein M, Atkins J, Barr H, Hammick M, Koppel I, Reeves S. A systematic review of interprofessional education. *Journal of Interprofessional Care* 1999; **13**: 417–24.
4. Owens P, Carrier J, Horder J. Interprofessional Issues in Community and Primary Health Care. London; Macmillan, 1995.
5. Soothill K, Mackay L, Webb C. *Interprofessional Relations in Health Care*. London: Edward Arnold, 1995.
6. CAIPE. Cultivating collaboration worldwide. www.caipe.org.uk, 2000. Accessed 11.11.00.
7. Department of Health. *A Health Service of all the Talents: Developing the NHS Workforce*. London: DoH, 2000.
8. Department of Health. *The NHS Plan: a Plan for Investment, a Plan for Reform*. London: DoH, 2000.
9. Burton J. Multipractice and Interprofessional learning in the community: a problem-based approach to improving cancer care. *Education for General Practice* 2000; **11**: 51–8.
10. Kirkpatrick D. Evaluation of training. In: Craig R, Bittel L, eds. *Training and Development Handbook*. New York: McGraw-Hill, 1967.
11. Klein R, Dixon J. Cash bonanza for NHS. *British Medical Journal* 2000; **320**: 883–4.
12. Barr H, Freeth M, Hammick M, Koppel I, Reeves S. *Evaluating Interprofessional Education*. London: CAIPE, 1999.
13. Burton J. Locality learning: from a lecture to a locality based specialist nurse: how did it happen? *CAIPE Bulletin* 1997; **13**: 27–8.
14. Burton J, Jackson N, McEwen Y. GP tutors, work-based learning and primary care groups. *Education for General Practice* 1999; **10**: 417–23.
15. Souster V. Tailor made training. *Journal of the Learning Workplace*. 1999; **Autumn/winter**: 2–7. (access through www.tlw.org.uk)
16. General Medical Council. *Teamworking in Medicine*. London: GMC, 2000.

17.   Wilson T, Mires G. A comparison of performance in medical and mid-
      wifery students in multi-professional teaching. *Medical Education* 2000;
      34: 744–6.

4 Clinical governance and education and training

MIKE PRINGLE AND
DAME LESLEY SOUTHGATE

Background and principles

Accountability

As we enter the third millennium, the accountability
of medical practitioners is national news in the United
Kingdom. The issues are complex, but we do well to
remember that they are essentially unchanged in many
respects from those that have been debated since the emergence of a recognizable medical profession. By the early
part of the nineteenth century, advances in physiology,
pathology, and chemistry were still not reflected in medical practice. In addition, there was widespread cynicism
amongst the general public, many of whom considered
doctors useless or dangerous, views based on observations
of the outcomes of treatments such as bleeding or purging
in the face of epidemics. In England there were opposing
views about the solution. Some favoured control by mandatory licensing, others advocated complete freedom of
choice for patients with anybody free to practise medicine.
These advocates of a free market argued that regulation
would lead to a self-serving restriction of others by the
medical profession. Then, as now, these events concerned
the profession, the public view of the effectiveness of medical practice and the trustworthiness of doctors, and the
government of the day through its law-making powers.

Eventually the Medical Act of 1858 formalized the body to which doctors must belong and empowered one organization, the General Medical Council, to regulate membership. Until the 1980s, the GMC concerned itself with behaviour that might undermine the reputation of the profession as a whole. Fraud, dishonesty, and the abuse of position were regarded with particular seriousness.

In essence this was a 'light touch' self-regulation of the profession in which clinical freedom was largely a matter of trust and the professional conscience, circumscribed by the GMC's action on more extreme cases of reported misbehaviour. It was supplemented by civil law cases for negligence—a rarely used but powerful mode of accountability—and Service Committee hearings. The latter concerned perceived deviation from the terms of the general practitioners' contract.

Modern professional regulation depends on a complex web of accountabilities being present and effective. The first—and probably most powerful—is the internal accountability to ourselves. Next, professionals such as doctors have traditionally been held to be accountable to peers. However, the accountability for GPs is much more complex and extends far beyond, while including, professional regulation. Any discussion of the interface between clinical governance and education and training must place our accountability into a broader framework.

To ourselves

The internal driver should not be underestimated. All health professionals are expected to aspire to deliver high quality of care and to recognize when they fall beneath acceptable standards. The edifice of education is based, and will continue to be based, on an internal imperative towards quality. All our aspirations for adult learning through continuing professional development are based on the assumption that doctors are aware of their limitations and motivated to correct them. Only the most cynical or sick doctor loses this insight, but for many the driver is insufficiently strong to achieve the continual improvement in care that peers and the public seek.

To our patients

GPs are also accountable to their patients as individuals. In the days before the National Health Service, patients directly represented income. Now the link between patient registrations and income is weaker. But individual patients can make the difference between a great day—a justified compliment can lift an entire surgery session onto a new plane—and a bad day, when a complaint or comment can too easily demoralize. We live for years with patients, sometimes our relationship coloured by one event many years earlier. Our reputations, so precious to us, can be made by word of mouth from a few patients. And patients can take their complaints into practice procedures, the primary care organization, the courts, or the General Medical Council.

To peers and colleagues

We are also accountable to our peers and colleagues. Others read our notes and consult with our patients. For single-handed doctors, the advent of out-of-hours cooperatives has offered a peer review group, sometimes for the first time. Practice clinical meetings, such as for significant event auditing[1] or conventional auditing, offer strong routes to peer accountability. Vocational trainers are used to being visited and reviewed by colleagues.

The Royal College of General Practitioners has a number of quality assurance programmes incorporating peer review. These include Fellowship by Assessment, Membership by Assessment of Performance, Accredited Professional Development, Quality Practice Award and Quality Team Development. And now primary care organizations, such as primary care trusts or groups, have clinical governance leaders who visit practices and look at systems and care delivered.

Through contract to our major employer, the NHS

Since the creation of the National Health Service in 1948, GPs have always been accountable to their major employer. This has been through a contract that has been a mixture of imperative and incentive. Tribunals and health authority procedures have acted on breaches of contract. In the past 2 years, clinical governance has become a statutory structure for local accountability within the NHS.[2]

The proposals in *Supporting Doctors, Protecting Patients*[3] may further change the nature of professionally led regulation. The policy of regular annual appraisal will either reinforce our professional processes—internal and peer— for quality or may impose a performance management framework that is more to do with compliance with NHS expectations than good professional activity.

By introducing the Postgraduate Education Allowance (PGEA) in 1989, the Department of Health crucially influenced the amount and nature of GP education. They have the same potential again, as the payment system is geared towards rewarding continuing professional development. Equally, the political expectation of personal development plans will drive educational behavioural change.[4]

To the profession in partnership with the public through professionally led regulation

The medical profession expects its members to be competent and it is supporting the introduction of revalidation, which is a process by which all registered practitioners will demonstrate that they are currently fit to practise. Collective pressure is exerted on individual colleagues to keep up to date, develop their care, and demonstrate their standards. The ultimate embodiment of this pressure is the General Medical Council and its procedures.

In recent decades, the General Medical Council has reacted to public and professional disquiet by introducing its processes for responding to problems deriving from a doctor's state of health in the 1980s. In the 1990s it introduced the performance procedures and for the first time became concerned directly with underperformance in clinical practice. As these reforms have been established, the proportion of lay members on the Council and participating in all of its activities has increased significantly.

Finally, GPs are accountable to the public and society. We are still trusted with decision making in sensitive and complex areas such as start-of-life decisions like termination of pregnancy, end-of-life decisions such as palliation, and all areas in between, including rationing. Society looks to doctors to be wise stabilizing forces and advisers and when disappointments and tragedies occur they are seen as a betrayal of trust.

Increasingly, GPs are becoming involved in wider health issues. At first it was lifestyle and risk behaviour, such as smoking, weight, diet, and exercise. Now it is increasingly environmental, as the links between housing and asthma, inequalities and mortality, employment and mental health, and pollution and disease all become evident. Society expects this role and is increasingly holding us to account for how effectively we deliver it.

So the starting thesis of this chapter is that GPs are accountable, not through one mechanism, but in multiple ways. They are accountable to themselves, their patients, their peers and colleagues, the NHS, their profession, and society at large. The importance of this for education and training is examined next.

Lifelong learning

To be effective, a GP must combine knowledge, skills, attitudes, and behaviour into achieving performance. The dimensions in which performance must occur are:

- technical knowledge and care, including use of best evidence;
- efficient use of resources;
- team working;
- access and availability;
- communication skills;
- ability to sustain long-term doctor–patient relationships;
- values of caring, honesty, and trust;
- advocacy for individual patients and communities.

The outcomes that are desired are good clinical outcomes for individuals and groups of patients; patient satisfaction and empowerment; and a contented coherent primary care team. Such an aspiration sees the GP achieving job satisfaction and personal health and contentment as a key contributor to these outcomes.

Given this job description—however idealized—it is then important to consider how it is achieved. The basic knowledge, skills, and attitudes can be set within the undergraduate experience. 'Finals' only measure these dimensions. Performance—in essence the application of knowledge, skills and attitudes—can only be learned, assessed, and promoted later.

Lifelong learning is therefore a portmanteau phrase for the processes that must occur throughout a GP's career to ensure good and improving performance. Some of the accountabilities already discussed are powerful drivers towards lifelong learning. Some are positive, reinforcing the internal desire to be a good doctor. Peer pressure and the need to be respected can be useful; patient comments, compliments, and criticisms are powerful; and rewards through contractual payment can be effective.

Some of the pressure to keep up to date comes from negative drivers. We all dread litigation and formal complaints. No doctor wants the shame of a General Medical Council hearing. These are increasingly serious influences on the educational motivation of doctors and must be recognized.

A formative review undertaken by a colleague can be a powerful method for encouraging lifelong learning. The insight that derives from an honest confidential discussion of strengths and weaknesses with an informed peer can set an agenda for personal development. Such an appraisal can work to maximize the positive drivers and lead to a personal development plan that is effective.

An assessment, however, that looks at performance against a range of indicators that are less about patient care than about cost and conformance, works on the negative level. The doctor will attempt to comply in order to avoid undesirable outcomes. Such appraisals would not lead to effective lifelong learning but to ritualistic activity designed to avoid painful effects.

As the culture shifts from loose to strong accountability, the balance between these positive and negative drivers will be crucial. If the primary care world becomes one of assessment and punishment, then continuing professional development will not flourish. If it is, in fact, based on a no-blame culture of quality assurance and improvement supporting lifelong development, then the outlook for patient care will be welcome.

So how does this relate to clinical governance? Primary care organizations have two main tasks within clinical governance. They must protect the public and foster improved care.[5] There is a responsibility to be confident that all doctors, nurses, and teams are not underperforming. Then the task is to facilitate the growth of those individuals and teams to ensure better care in the future.

Quality assurance

Clinical audit can be seen as a mechanical activity undertaken to meet contractual requirement or to achieve payment. This was the philosophy instilled by the 1989 reforms. Its links to education and training were regarded as tenuous and secondary.

We now recognize that the collection of facts or case descriptions in abstract is not linked to either change in care or personal development. Both of the latter processes are emotional primarily, but built on an intellectual understanding of the requirement. A table of data can be assimilated intellectually, but only achieves change when it is linked to an emotional context. Box 4.1 illustrates this.

The concept of a personal development plan is that reflection and awareness can be linked to the identification of educational needs and thus meeting them. This, in turn, leads to better patient care, a more rounded doctor and/or development of services. Box 4.1 illustrates one method of developing awareness of education need. There

---

Box 4.1   Quality assurance and educational need

The practice had been auditing its care of diabetes for many years. Every year the computer records were analysed and a range of indicators compiled. These were published in the practice report and were widely available. Over the years the percentage of patients with diabetes recorded as having their eyes examined for retinopathy within the past 14 months was reasonably constant at just over 50%.

Nobody in the practice team was happy about this. Discussions were repeated every year and focused around the completeness of recording. Since most patients went to an optician for their eye check, it was all too easy for these data not to be entered by the doctor or nurse during the person with diabetes' annual review.

The practice also had significant event auditing meetings every month. At these meetings the doctors, nurses, other clinical staff, and managers discussed the care of individual patients. These might include a young man with a myocardial infarction, a girl with an unplanned pregnancy or a new diagnosis of cancer. Such discussions often reveal good care and result in congratulations. However, some such discussions reveal shortcomings that need to be corrected.

One such discussion concerned an 83-year-old lady who was in residential care and who had been registered blind with diabetic retinopathy. The notes revealed that she had not had an annual diabetes review for 6 years since she was unable to attend the surgery. She had no review of her retina recorded except for one doctor recording many years ago 'fundi ✓'. The doctor concerned expressed concerns that he might not be as confident in retinal screening as he was, since he did so little of it now.

After lengthy discussion the team decided:

continued

- to institute annual visits for diabetic checks for those people with diabetes in residential and nursing homes;
- to explore with a local optician the possibility of retinal screening for these people;
- for the doctors to have a session updating their fundoscopy skills.

Years of conventional audits had resulted in hand wringing. One case led to the identification of process issues, team work problems, and educational need.

are many others. Regular peer appraisal is one; team-based discussion is another. Multidisciplinary learning has helped some to develop their awareness.

The introduction of video-recording for vocational trainer assessment and for summative assessment was, for many doctors, a key way to see themselves as others see them, and to develop self-awareness. Patient questionnaires, interviews, and focus groups can offer similar insights.

The key to quality assurance feeding into the educational agenda is the individual's willingness to develop self-awareness and to act on it. The enemies are complacency and denial. So clinical governance should primarily be asking teams about the ways in which they promote insight and awareness; how they support each other to meet their education needs; and how they ensure that lessons learned are implemented in the day-to-day work of the practice.

However, there is the element of clinical governance that must ensure the protection of the public. A primary care organization must ensure that any problems that it identifies—such as outlying prescribing or referring behaviour—is looked at and, if appropriate, addressed. It must be sure that systems to identify underperformance are in place and are effective, and that action to remedy poor performance is undertaken. This is the other face of education and training.

Remedial action

As a profession we are more comfortable promoting continuous improvement than acting to address failing colleagues. Partly this is avoidance of difficult tasks—many underperforming doctors lack insight into their problems and resist effective solutions. Partly it is because we prefer not to look into the black night of failure, of patients at risk, and of professional vulnerability. And partly it is because we find it difficult to distinguish personal underperformance from that of systems.

It is easy to have sympathy for a single-handed doctor in a highly deprived area coping with a large registered list. The premises are poor and the support team almost non-existent. She says she is trying her best but delivering good care requires superhuman abilities.

Nobody wants to blame that individual GP for their environment. Yet, we know that other similar practices have not opted for a large list/low service model, but have reasonable numbers of patients. Premises and staffing levels are under the control of the GPs. Many practices do deliver good care in deprived areas—it is just more difficult to do than in affluent areas.

Distinguishing the 'system' from the 'individuals' will always be difficult. Performance indicators seldom tell us the true picture.[6] So just as self-awareness is a key to personal learning, local awareness is vital to understanding the development needs of individuals, teams, and systems.

Once, however, poor care is found, there is an obligation to act. For years GPs in any area have known of individual colleagues and practices that were underperforming. It was not their problem. They looked to the health authority and the health authority looked to the Local Medical Committee which in turn looked to the General Medical Council. In this 'pass the parcel' nobody addressed the real issues.

Now it is everybody's business. One key outcome of the Bristol paediatric cardiothoracic surgery case is that a medically qualified manager was held to account for not acting on the alleged underperformance of others.[7] All doctors must act if they have sufficient grounds for suspecting underperformance.

And the chief executives of primary care trusts have a statutory obligation to act to protect the public from poor performance.[8] Increasingly, as the General Medical Council tightens up its processes, the care delivered by all doctors is becoming everybody's business.

Once poor performance is found, there are several next steps. The first is to examine the systems. If the doctor has been asking for support but has been denied the tools to do their job, then the managers and local primary care organizations must be held to account. If the problem is poor organization and practice management, then that must be addressed.

If, however, the problem is one of poor knowledge, skills, or attitudes feeding into poor performance, then this is an educational task. It requires a full diagnostic process, agreed educational needs, support, intervention, reassessment, and long-term mentoring and facilitation. This is no mean agenda.

Traditionally educational provision in the United Kingdom has been geared to addressing higher needs. We have no provision at present for effectively picking up a failed GP and putting intensive support in place to ensure a revived career. In time regular appraisal and revalidation may ensure that GPs who are failing will be detected at an early stage and encouraged to resume their personal development. That may reduce the scale of our task. But it will not eradicate it.

The Chief Medical Officer has proposed an Assessment and Support Service to perform the tasks described here in handling underperforming doctors.[3,9] This cannot be a service divorced from the educational processes for other doctors, from GP tutors and directors, from the deaneries. However, few doctors would relish having an under-performing colleague in their practice having intensive supervision and re-education. Developments in remedial support will be fascinating to watch, and difficult to deliver, over the next few years.

Examples of practical application

One of the unifying forces in a bewildering array of lines of accountability for the modern GP is the General Medical Council's guidance, *Good Medical Practice*. This generic guidance on what will be expected from every registered doctor will form the basis for determining the curriculum for education and training throughout medicine. It provides an expanded definition of modern practice to include relationships with patients, teamwork, participation in continuing professional development, and a commitment to maintaining performance placed alongside the traditional competency in diagnosis, management, and practical skills that make up good clinical care. It applies from entry to medical school right through to retirement.

Revalidation for clinical general practice

Revalidation might be thought, at first, to have little connection to 'education'. The General Medical Council has decreed that revalidation will occur for all doctors at regular intervals to confirm their fitness to practise. It is therefore a minimum performance test that should be more about meeting performance criteria than education, lifelong learning, and personal development. It is however an 'assessment' and by definition becomes a powerful driver for learning.

Each doctor will be revalidated against *Good Medical Practice*. The statements in this document include those in Box 4.2.

Because this is still a very generic statement, the Royal College of General Practitioners created a working group, under the chairmanship of Professor Martin Roland, to look at the implications of these statements for GPs. The resulting document, *Good Medical Practice for General Practitioners*, gives specific statement concerning the unacceptable GP (see Box 4.3). These will be used as the basis for revalidation for GPs.

Clearly, the criteria for revalidation will include effective educational activity. Further, revalidation is seen as a continuous process with an episodic, 5-year review. Each year every GP will have a peer appraisal that is in essence formative and educational. However, the summative outcome will be a signed statement by the appraiser that the appraisal has properly occurred, that the appraisee is on route to revalidation (in other words has a folder in preparation) and that no evidence of underperformance has been identified.

Those GPs experiencing difficulties with meeting the standards of revalidation will need to be supported through an analysis of the problems and addressing solutions.

Box 4.2   *Good Medical Practice*, paragraphs 5, 6, and 7

You must keep your knowledge and skills up to date throughout your working life. In particular, you should take part regularly in educational activities which develop your competence and performance

You must work with colleagues to monitor and maintain your awareness of the quality of the care you provide. In particular, you must:

- take part in regular and systematic medical and clinical audit, recording data honestly. Where necessary you must respond to the results of audit to improve your practice, for example by undertaking further training;
- respond constructively to assessments and appraisals of your professional competence and performance.

Some parts of medical practice are governed by law or are regulated by other statutory bodies. You must observe and keep up to date with the laws and statutory codes of practice which affect your work.

If these solutions are educational, then the challenge for the educational establishment is clear.

Revalidation is primarily about protecting and assuring the public. It must reliably detect and address unacceptable levels of performance. However, it will act as the platform from which lifelong learning can develop. By bringing all GPs into contact with mentors, appraisers, and educationalists, revalidation should establish the infrastructure and culture to ensure effective continuing professional development and lifelong learning.

Box 4.3   The relevant attributes, which are not exhaustive, for an unacceptable general practitioner in *Good Medical Practice for General Practitioners*

- has little knowledge of developments in clinical practice
- has limited insight into the current state of his or her knowledge or performance
- selects educational events which do not reflect his or her learning needs
- does not audit care in his or her practice, or does not feed the results back into practice
- is hostile to external audit or advice
- does not understand or respond to the law relating to general practice
- where employing staff, neither understands nor meets his or her responsibilities as an employer
- has unsafe premises, e.g. hazardous chemicals or sharp instruments are inadequately protected

Accredited Professional Development

The Royal College of General Practitioners will be launching Accredited Professional Development in 2001. This is a continuous scheme whereby participating GPs will be able to demonstrate that their professional development is of a good standard. It will also over a 5-year period include all the activities required for revalidation, set out under the headings of *Good Medical Practice*. This then is a scheme that will allow GPs to fulfil their personal development plans, to meet the requirements of clinical governance, to gain any payments for continuing professional development that may be introduced, and to satisfy the requirements of revalidation. It is set significantly above the minimum expectations of revalidation, but at a level that all competent GPs should find possible. Programmes such as these will enable the competent majority to achieve revalidation through programmes that are stimulating, enjoyable, and encouraging, thereby avoiding the negativity and demoralization that can come from fulfilling minimum standards only.

It is intended that Membership by Assessment of Performance and Fellowship by Assessment will also be approved as evidence to satisfy the requirements of revalidation. However, since these two systems do not include regular appraisal, they will need to be supplemented by annual appraisal certificates. Accredited Professional Development includes annual appraisal and will be a complete revalidation package in its own right.

The General Medical Council's Performance Procedures

If a GP is performing poorly and local efforts to identify and remedy the causes are unsuccessful, then referral to the GMC fitness to practise procedures will follow. In the future doctors who are not recommended for revalidation will also automatically be referred. If poor health or misconduct are ruled out by the screener, the GP will be referred into the Performance Procedures. The content of the assessment is also based on *Good Medical Practice*. However, because the consequences for a GP's career can be very serious, the assessment is rigorous and very detailed and includes all the areas relevant to the pattern of poor performance raised by the complaints to the Council. It is usually held over 3 days for a GP, 2 days at the doctor's practice followed by 1 day of tests of knowledge and skills at a test centre. The process is described in detail here because it demonstrates the range of assessments that are used, some of which may in simpler versions be relevant to collecting evidence for revalidation. The elements of the programme are similar to other programmes for assessing performance around the world.[10]

Planning the peer review visit

The peer review of performance is carried out over 2 days, at the site of actual practice, by two medical assessors and one lay assessor. The purpose of the visit is to enable the assessors to review a reasonable sample of the whole of the doctor's clinical practice and to compare it with the standards expressed in *Good Medical Practice* and elaborated within the RCGP document *Good Medical Practice for General Practitioners*.

Each visit is planned using a standard portfolio, in which the doctor describes his/her training, experience, and circumstances of practice. The document also provides an opportunity for doctors to rate their familiarity and confidence in dealing with common and important general practice problems and to self-assess their own communication skills. GPs are asked to submit their most recent prescribing catalogue. The doctor is encouraged to fill it in with the help of an advisor.

The portfolio also serves another important purpose. Through it the doctor presents to the assessors the implicit standard at which he or she claims to practice. The doctor tells the assessors what sort of doctor he/she is and what is the content of actual practice The assessors use this information to define what they can reasonably expect of this doctor when they visit the workplace.

Medical record keeping

The assessment of medical record keeping allows the assessors to examine the structure and content of the doctor's records in relation to predefined criteria. There are explicit guidelines for the selection of the records to ensure that an adequate number and range are inspected. Medical record keeping is assessed in its own right, it is not regarded as a surrogate for other aspects of the doctor's performance, such as clinical reasoning, which are assessed elsewhere in the procedures.[11]

Case-based oral

Case-based orals (chart-stimulated recall) are a powerful means of assessing clinical performance[12] and during an assessment doctors discuss their own cases with the medical assessors. Judgements are documented against criteria of acceptable and unacceptable performance, which direct the discussion to aspects of practice similar to those identified in other programmes where fitness to practise is at issue. These include quality of clinical reasoning, recognizing the limits of your own competence, when to refer, and prescribing.[13] The medical assessors conduct the discussion but some cases are also assessed by the lay assessor to judge the way that the doctor talked about his/her patient.

Observation of aspects of actual practice

The assessors observe consultations with patients. The patient is asked for informed consent for the medical or sometimes the lay assessor to be present. A generic instrument allows the assessors to record a judgement about the doctor-centred and patient-centred aspects of the consultation.[14] Concerns about the doctor's knowledge base or clinical method can be raised by the assessors during the case-based oral or the interview with the doctor.

Site tour and interview

For those doctors who have a direct responsibility for the standard of the premises and equipment and for practice organization, the assessment will include a judgement about whether those things that can reasonably be expected by patients, and which are in the control of the doctor, are in place. There is evidence that aspects of practice management, such as the availability of essential equipment, is related to performance with patients.[15] The lay assessor conducts this aspect of the assessment. The site tour is recorded in a structured way. Informal conversations are discouraged, with the opportunity to clarify or discuss made available in the formal interview sessions.

Third party interviews

Interviews with those who regularly work with the doctor concerned are an important part of the peer review visit. Other similar programmes also place a high value on the views of colleagues for the assessment of clinical performance.[16-18] The validity of the interviews comes from the GMC's guidance, *Good Medical Practice*, on which they are based. The format is the same for the entire profession. Interviews are conducted with at least two assessors present, chaired by the lay assessor, and are recorded verbatim by a shorthand writer. At least 12 people are interviewed, five of whom can be nominated by the doctor. A family doctor's colleagues might include, for example, other doctors in the practice, including doctors in training, practice nurses, midwives, health visitors, pharmacist, administrators, and the consultant in the local A&E department.

Structured interview with the doctor and concluding meeting of the assessors

The final assessment in the peer review visit takes the form of a structured interview conducted by the whole panel. The assessment panel meets before the interview to review their findings so far and to plan the agenda. The lay assessor chairs the session and the doctor is entitled to have a supporter with him or her. No feedback is given as the assessors still have to consider all the information and make a decision about whether to proceed to phase 2 tests of competence which will include a knowledge test, a simulated surgery, and a test of practical skills.

Reporting the assessment to the Council

At the conclusion of the assessment, the lead assessor writes a report for the GMC case coordinator. It includes a judgement about effects of circumstances of practice on the doctor's performance.

The report goes on to compare the doctor's practice with the standards of *Good Medical Practice*. For each category, the assessors decide whether the doctor's performance is: 'acceptable', 'cause for concern', or 'unacceptable'.[19] Both strengths and weaknesses are addressed. No-one is perfect and we have found 'cause for concern' in some aspect of every doctor's performance. All of the independent judgements made over the 2 days of the peer review visit, with supporting evidence, are collated to the headings within *Good Medical Practice* to which they refer. Assessors weigh the evidence using the principles of triangulation; they must corroborate evidence from at least three sources before making a judgement. In practice, 500–700 independent judgements are recorded during a peer review. More than 25 GPs had been assessed by the end of 2000. Some of them were not performing poorly when they were visited, and all these doctors went on to do well in the tests. In several cases the quality of the local documentation of the complaint and the approach to local resolution and remediation was considered by the GMC assessors to be very poor. This finding highlights the need for coordination of local efforts, good management, and training for those who are engaged in identifying and supporting doctors who are struggling. The missing piece of the jigsaw should be the NCCA, provided its remit is to support and not to punish.

References

1. Pringle M, Bradley C. Significant event auditing: a user's guide. *Audit Trends* 1994; **2**(1): 20–3.
2. Department of Health. *A First Class Service—Quality in the New NHS*. London: Department of Health, 1998.
3. Department of Health. *Supporting Doctors, Protecting Patients*. London: Department of Health, 1999.
4. Chief Medical Officer. *A Review of Continuing Professional Development in General Practice*. London: Department of Health, 1998.
5. RCGP. *Clinical Governance in General Practice*. London: RCGP, 1998.
6. RCGP. *Recognising Quality of Care in General Practice*. London: RCGP, 1998.
7. Smith R. All changed, changed utterly. *British Medical Journal* 1998; **316**: 1917–18.
8. Department of Health. *The New NHS: Modern and Dependable*. London: Department of Health, 1997.
9. Department of Health. *The NHS Plan*. London: Department of Health, 2000.
10. Page G, Bates J, Dyer S, *et al*. Physician-assessment and physician-enhancement programs in Canada. *Canadian Medical Association Journal* 1995; **153**(12): 1723–8.
11. Rethans J-J, Martin E, Metsemakers J. To what extent do clinical notes by general practitioners reflect actual medical performance? A study using simulated patients. *British Journal of General Practice* 1994; **44**: 153–6.

12. Solomon D, Reinhart M, Bridgham R, *et al.* An assessment of an oral examination format for evaluating clinical competence in emergency medicine. *Academic Medicine* 1990; **65**: 9.

13. Miller F, Jacques A, Brailovsky C, Sindon A, Bordage G. When to recommend compulsory versus optional CME programs? *Academic Medicine* 1997; **72**(9): 760–4.

14. Levenstein J, McCracken E, McWhinney I, Stewart M, Brown J. The patient-centered clinical method 1. A model for the doctor–patient interaction in family medicine. *Family Practice* 1986; **3**: 24–30.

15. Ram P, Grol R, van den Hombergh P, Rethans JJ, van den Vleuten C, Aretz K. Structure and process: the relationship between practice management and actual clinical performance in general practice. *Family Practice* 1998; **15**(4): 354–62.

16. Ramsey P, Weinrich M. Use of professional associate ratings to assess the performance of practising physicians: past, present, future. *Advances in Health Science Education* 1999; **4**: 27–38.

17. Newble D, Paget N. The evaluation of the Practice Quality Review component of the Maintenance of Professional Standards program in the RACP. In: Scherpbier A, van der Vleuten C, Rethans J, van der Steeg A, eds. *Advances in Medical Education*. Dordrecht: Kluwer Academic, 1997: 567–70.

18. Ramsey P, Wenrich C, Inui T, Larson E, LoGerfo J. Use of peer ratings to evaluate physician performance. *Journal of the American Medical Association* 1993; **269**: 1655–60.

19. Southgate L, Cox J, Hatch D, Johnson N, Jolly B. The assessment of poorly performing doctors: the development of the assessment methods for the General Medical Council's Performance Procedures. Submitted for publication.

5 The principles of educational support in primary care

JOHN SPENCER

Introduction

Education and training, and the ability to manage change successfully lie at the heart of the future development of general practice and primary care. Traditional models of continuing education and professional development will need to change significantly in the face of the new challenges. Clinical governance, personal and practice development plans, revalidation, evidence-based practice, and multiprofessional working all demand a different philosophy and approach to learning.

Effective learning and change management are underpinned by a number of important ideas, many supported by a growing evidence base.[1] Some of these will be covered in this chapter, namely:

- adult learners, self-directed learning, and the learning environment;
- learning styles;
- problem-based learning and evidence-based practice;
- experiential learning, reflective practice, and task-based education;
- feedback, appraisal, assessment, and evaluation;
- mentoring;
- groups, teams, and multiprofessional learning;

- managing change.

Examples of particular educational approaches and tools supported by these principles are described, along with suggestions for further reading. Finally, some of the specific challenges relating to education in primary care are discussed.

Adult learners, self-directed learning, and the learning environment

Ideas about the 'adult learner' are based on five assumptions:[2]

- as they mature, people become less dependent and more self-directed, thus more capable of determining their own learning needs and finding ways to meet them;
- experience is a rich resource for learning;
- an adult's readiness to learn is closely related to tasks facing them in their work and they value learning immediately relevant to those tasks;
- adults value learning that can be put into practice immediately; and
- motivation to learn comes as much from internal as from external influences.

Self-directed learning

The concept of self-directed learning (SDL) underpins many theories of learning, notably adult learning.[3] In SDL the learner takes initiative for their own learning, diagnosing learning needs, formulating goals and objectives, identifying resources, implementing appropriate activities, and evaluating outcomes. SDL has been suggested as the most efficacious approach for the continuum of health-care education, and the one most likely to produce health-care professionals prepared for lifelong learning, able to meet the changing needs of the service and their patients.[4]

SDL is an active process, encouraging adoption of a so-called 'deep approach' to learning. Deep learning involves an active search for meaning. The learner is motivated by interest in the subject and by its vocational relevance, their goal being to reach an understanding of the material. By contrast, learners adopting a 'surface approach' are predominantly driven by concern to complete the course or pass an examination, or by fear of failure. The outcome is superficial understanding. Implicit to the concept of SDL is acceptance of personal responsibility for learning, which itself requires the learner to have genuine choice and a large degree of autonomy. Finally, self-directed learners need feedback on their performance.

The concept of the 'adult learner' has been challenged, partly because it is based on the assumption that people are effective in identifying their own learning needs. Unfortunately, evidence in respect of the latter is not good, certainly if learners are left to their own devices.[5]

One problem is the tendency to identify 'wants' (driven by personal choice and interest) rather than 'needs'. This may be overcome by using methods that attempt to identify areas of real need. One research and development project into continuing professional development (CPD) identified no fewer than 48 such methods,[6] focused on six areas of practice:

- clinician's experience (e.g. PUNs and DENs—see later);
- interactions within the team (e.g. meetings);
- non-clinical activities (e.g. journal articles);
- formal approaches to quality management (e.g. clinical audit);

- specific needs assessment activities (e.g. significant event analysis—see later);
- peer review (e.g. appraisal—see later).

PUNs and DENs

This is a good example of a simple way of identifying educational needs, although it has only been subjected to limited evaluation.[7] The two acronyms stand for 'patients' unmet needs' and 'doctors' educational needs'. The doctor identifies a PUN by asking the question 'Was I equipped to meet the patient's needs?', and defines the DEN by asking 'Could I have done better?'. Documentation in the form of a diary or logbook is required. Strengths of the method are that it is cheap, requires minimum time and effort, is relevant to the work of busy practitioners, can identify both individual education and training, as well as practice development needs, and is linked to improvement in patient care. The main weaknesses are that it still requires effort to define a PUN or DEN (which may not be immediately apparent), it does not guarantee that unmet needs will be addressed, and the *patient's* needs are defined by the doctor.

Learning environment

The term 'learning environment' describes the overall educational climate. It encompasses a wide range of factors, including the underlying 'culture' (how much learning is valued and supported), relationships between teachers and learners, the nature of the tasks, the resources provided, methods of assessment, and physical factors, to name a few. It is regarded as one of the most important factors in motivation, and some theorists have argued that getting it right is the most important thing an educator can do. An environment conducive to learning is one which:

• is supportive and safe;
• fosters collaboration and cooperation;
• values the contributions of individuals;
• is based on mutual respect.

Various strategies for creating a supportive environment have been described. For example, Gibb identified six categories of behaviour characteristic of supportive situations, which could be consciously employed to develop such a climate. These are predominantly attitudinal or interpersonal, rather than organizational factors.[8] Maslow, on the other hand, described a hierarchy of needs. At the very basic level, the learners' physiological and physical needs must be met. Next, come emotional and social needs. Only then, he argued, can higher order needs such as learning and problem solving be addressed.[9]

Putting together these ideas, we can conclude that adults will be motivated by learning characterized by certain features, as shown in Box 5.1.

Three broad categories of SDL for clinicians have been described:

• informal activities, often ad hoc, such as journal reading, discussions with colleagues, interactions with pharmaceutical representatives;
• semi-structured activities, usually focused on patient or practice problems that require an immediate solution; and
• formal planned SDL, where there is a clear intention to learn about a particular issue.

It can be seen that the traditional model of CME (the lunchtime lecture given by a specialist on 'Latest advances in . . . .' to a group of general practitioners reluctantly fulfilling statutory requirements for postgraduate education allowance) is in almost every way the antithesis of the 'adult learner' approach.

Box 5.1   Principles of adult learning

Adults will be motivated by learning which:

- is relevant to their present working situation
- takes account of, and builds on, their previous experience
- is directed towards their perceived needs
- involves them in planning
- enables them to diagnose their own needs
- is practical, rather than theoretical, and is focused on real-life problems
- actively involves them and is geared to their own style and pace of learning
- is designed so they can take responsibility for their own learning
- promotes an atmosphere conducive to learning
- involves them in evaluation through self- and peer assessment.

This has been confirmed in a number of systematic reviews of the efficacy of CME, and methods of changing doctors' behaviour.[10,11] Interventions least likely to produce change are one-off events, unsolicited dissemination of materials, didactic lectures, and passive participation. Change is more likely, however, when there has been a needs assessment, when education is linked to practise, when motivation for participation involves some personal incentive, and when there are reinforcing features. Single interventions more likely to be effective include:

- individualized audit feedback;
- advice from a respected colleague;
- a visit by a non-commercial adviser (so-called 'educational outreach'); and
- patient-mediated interventions with reminders.

Multi-faceted approaches are more likely to work than single ones, and indeed most interventions are effective under some circumstances. Unfortunately,none is effective under all circumstances. There are no magic bullets![11]

Learning styles

Whereas learners use different approaches according to circumstances, individual learning *style* is thought to be a more stable phenomenon. The concept of 'learning style' has been viewed from a number of perspectives, the differences stemming largely from underlying theoretical frameworks. As with any attempt to classify human behaviour, there are limitations to all models. One of the commoner classifications is derived from management studies by Honey and Mumford.[12] Scores from an 80-item questionnaire are plotted onto a graph with four axes. This gives a visual representation of a person's individual learning style with reference to four different dimensions:

- activist—learns by doing and working with others, thrives on challenge and new experiences, dislikes being passive (*'What's new? I'm game for anything!'*);
- reflector—learns unhurriedly through thought and careful review; dislikes pressure (*'I'd like time to think this through'*);
- theorist—learns using theoretical models and concepts, through questioning and logic; dislikes inadequate information or ambiguity (*'How does 'this' relate to 'that'?'*); and
- pragmatist—prefers learning in a context where theory and practice are clearly linked (*'How can I apply this in practice?'*).

Everyone has elements of all these dimensions in varying degrees. Understanding their own style may help learners develop more effective ways of tackling learning.

Problem-based learning and evidence-based practice

Problem-based learning

First introduced into medical education at McMasters University in Ontario in the late 1960s, problem-based learning (PBL) has been described as one of the most significant developments in professional education, with around 10% of medical schools world wide and many other health-care education institutions having adopted it. There is no universal definition of PBL, the term being used to describe both an educational method and a curricular philosophy.

Nevertheless, PBL is generally understood to mean a process in which learners identify issues raised by specific problems to help develop understanding about underlying concepts. New knowledge and understanding arise from working on the problem, in contrast to traditional approaches in which new knowledge is a *prerequisite* for tackling the problem. It is usually a group activity and follows a particular sequence, such as the Maastricht 'seven jump', named after a Dutch children's song. The steps in this sequence are:

1　clarify terms and concepts;
2　define the problem(s) and agree which phenomena need explanation;
3　analyse the problem (usually by 'brainstorm');
4　develop working hypotheses and explanations;

5   generate and prioritize learning objectives;
6   research learning objectives (usually through inde-
    pendent study);
7   report back, synthesize explanations, and apply newly
    acquired information.

Generally, steps 1–5 are undertaken in an initial group
session, step 6 involves independent enquiry, often over a
period of time, and step 7 is dealt with at a further group
session.[13,14]

PBL is underpinned by the principles of SDL. It also concords with findings of cognitive psychology about learning,[15] in that it:

•   'activates prior knowledge' (a powerful starting point,
    given that learning builds on what the learner already
    knows);
•   motivates (through learning things in context);
•   promotes elaboration of knowledge (learning is an
    active process, in which meaning is generated by inter-
    play between new information and existing concepts);
•   fosters an inquisitive style (and thus a deep approach
    to learning).

PBL in undergraduate education has been extensively
researched, and there is a rich literature on the subject. Its
benefits and limitations are reasonably well understood.[16]
However, there are few descriptions of its use in postgraduate education.[17] Since one of its main benefits is fostering
group and interpersonal skills, it is argued that PBL would
be an ideal method for multiprofessional education.

Evidence-based practice

The ability to find and appraise evidence is obviously a
crucial skill in PBL, and it should be no surprise that the

evidence-based medicine, or 'evidence-based practice' model also emerged from McMasters. Evidence-based practice (EBP) has been proposed as a means of closing the gap between research and practice, and ensuring that clinical decisions are based on best available evidence. It has been defined as 'the conscientious, explicit and judicious use of current best evidence in making decisions about the care of individual patients',[18] and involves five steps, similar to PBL:

- identify the clinical question(s) to be investigated;
- track down the best evidence to answer them;
- critically appraise the evidence for validity (closeness to the truth) and usefulness (clinical applicability);
- apply the findings in clinical practice;
- evaluate performance.

Unfortunately, powerful though the imperative is, many health professionals may not possess the skills to practice EBP effectively and confidently. These include:

- framing the clinical question(s);
- searching for evidence (usually using electronic media—this requires working knowledge of available sources of evidence and how they are organized, as well as how to operate the searching software); and
- critically appraising the evidence.

However, many courses teaching EBP are now available, often based on the model developed by Sackett and colleagues in Oxford.[19] Unsurprisingly, such courses appear to be most successful when based on principles of adult, self-directed learning, although there is, as yet, little evidence that sustained change in learners' practice behaviours or patient outcomes results.

Experiential learning, reflective practice, and task-based education

Learning by doing: experiential learning and reflective practice

We all 'learn by doing', yet although experience creates powerful learning opportunities, it is not the entire source of learning. Particularly in the context of work-based learning, practice (experience or 'doing') needs to be linked to theory (underlying concepts) and this happens through the process of reflection. Several models of experiential learning have been described,[20] the common theme being the concept of a cyclical process linking concrete experience (doing) with abstract conceptualization (thinking), via reflection and experimentation, as in Figure 5.1.

The cycle can be 'entered' at any point, although usually via concrete experience. Wherever it is entered, learning will be most effective if the learner can move through all the stages and complete it. This requires a conducive learning environment in which an individual's experience

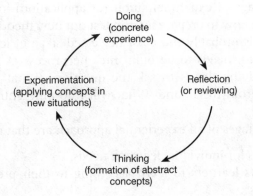

Figure 5.1   The experiential learning cycle (from Kolb[21]).

is valued, and there is support and structure for learning.

Reflection is standing back and thinking about an experience. It happens automatically, but in the hurly-burly of a busy working day, often only fleetingly. Learning will be more profound if reflection can become conscious, and as such it needs to be built into the learning cycle. It has been defined as:

paying deliberate, systematic and analytical attention to one's own actions, feelings and thinking in relation to particular experiences, for the purposes of retaining perceptions of, and responses to current and future experience.[22]

The process involves not only describing experience (What happened?), but also analysing and evaluating it (What does it mean? How does it relate to previous experience?), as well as attending to the feelings evoked (How did I feel?). It has been shown to be an effective tool in raising awareness of professionals to the wealth of learning in everyday practice, enabling practitioners to examine their actions, reasoning, and feelings, and hence to become more skilful and effective. Reflection can be promoted through reading, discussion, or writing.

The stage of experimentation (or application) involves planning how to prepare for and test out new theories and skills. It is probably the most neglected stage of learning and, again, needs to be built into the process. A simple way of doing this is to ask the questions 'What have I learned from this?', and 'What will I do differently next time?'.

Advantages of an experiential approach are that it:

- caters for individual learning needs;
- allows learners to learn according to their preferred styles;
- motivates because learning is shaped around experi-

ence;
- allows flexibility; and
- enables learners to build on what they already know.

The complexity of most learning situations, particularly in clinical practice, means that learners at any time may be engaged in several parallel cycles, with different time scales and at different stages. This begs the need for record keeping to keep track of the process.

Task-based learning

Task-based learning brings together the problem-based approach and experiential learning.[23] Everyday tasks provide the context, and learning is built around them. There are potential outcomes in several areas:

- learning about the task itself;
- in-depth understanding of a particular area;
- development of transferable knowledge and skills; and
- general competencies.

Other terms applied to this approach include 'service-based learning' and 'practice-based learning'.[20] Its particular appeal is that it is rooted in the learner's day-to-day experience, helping to make it effective, efficient, and relevant. It has been claimed it can thus resolve the potential conflict between service and training, and is also an appropriate approach when time available for formal education is limited.

Assessment, feedback, appraisal, and evaluation

These concepts are all inter-related, but can be confused, not least because the terms are used in different ways in different contexts, often interchangeably. They all share common features, however, not least that they are all ways of helping 'close the loop' of learning.

Assessment

It is impossible to overestimate the importance of assessment in the educational process.[24] It is one of the most important influences on learning, not only what is learned but also how it is learned. This principle is often lamented ('the tail that wags the dog') but can be exploited effectively. Assessment can be defined as a systematic procedure for measuring a sample of learners' thinking or behaviour in order to make a judgement about them. Assessment serves many purposes, ranging from measuring academic achievement to predicting future performance, each of which demands different things of the process, and particularly of the respective assessment instrument(s) used.

An assessment procedure can be either 'formative' or 'summative'. A *formative* assessment is intended to provide the learner with feedback on progress to help identify strengths and redirect learning towards areas of weakness. It should be an informal, on-going process forming an integral part of teaching and learning.[25] On the other hand, *summative* assessment is formal and usually occurs at the end of a prescribed period of instruction. It requires learners to demonstrate the 'sum' of their knowledge and skills, and its purpose is usually to decide about progress or certification. Formative tests ask the question 'How am I doing?'; summative tests ask 'How did I do?'. When, in addition to a mark or grade, feedback is given as part of a summative process, it may also be formative. Historically in medical education, at both undergraduate and postgraduate levels, despite a growing understanding of its 'technology', assessment has been heavily influenced by prejudice, hunch, and ignorance. Paradoxically, assessment is probably the area of education for which there is the most robust evidence base.

Unfortunately, in the measurement of clinical competence, there is no perfect assessment instrument.[23] The challenge is to approximate assessment to the real world, whilst maintaining standardized test conditions at a level appropriate to the learner. It is useful to consider the 'utility', or usefulness, of an assessment instrument as a (non-arithmetic) product of several factors:[26] validity, reliability, acceptability, cost, and educational impact.

Utility = Validity × Reliability × Acceptability × Cost × Educational Impact

- Validity—does it measure what it is supposed to measure?
- Reliability—does it consistently measure what it is supposed to measure?
- Acceptability—is it acceptable to all parties?
- Cost—what are the costs, including time and human resources?
- Educational impact—how will it drive learning?

All assessment instruments have advantages and disadvantages, and there is usually a trade-off between elements in the 'utility' equation.

Feedback

Learning is enhanced when we know how well we are doing; learners need feedback to learn effectively, so much so that it has been described as 'the life-blood of learning'. Unfortunately, feedback in medical education has historically often been either non-existent, or worse still, negative and destructive, rather than affirming and constructive, with a predictably inhibitory effect on learning.

Two practical approaches to feedback have emerged from communications skills teaching. The commonest model was described by Pendleton and colleagues, and has come to be known as 'Pendleton's rules'.[27] Essential features are discussion of positive issues first, self-assessment, and recommendations, not criticisms. The usual sequence is as follows:

- clarify matters of fact (to avoid misunderstandings);
- the learner then says what was done well, and how;
- the facilitator, and other group members if present, then comment on what was done well;
- the learner then says what could have been done differently, and how;
- the rest of the group then say what they feel could be done differently.

This approach has played an important role in medical education and, in the opinion of many, continues to be the most appropriate approach for situations in which learner, facilitator, and other group members do not know each other, or have not worked together before. However, certain potential difficulties that may limit the effectiveness of the method have been highlighted. These include:

- the artificiality of the process;
- the potential for evaluative and judgmental comments inherent in the notion of 'good and bad';

- the learner's agenda is discovered only late in the process; and
- there is inefficient use of time, in that disproportionate amounts may be spent on what worked well, with little left for constructive help with difficulties.

All in all, the process can seem contrived, even patronizing, particularly when a learner knows full well there have been problems, and wishes to address them.

An alternative approach that tackles some of these areas is the so-called 'agenda-led outcomes-based' approach.[8] It builds on the strengths of the above method, but goes 'straight for the jugular' by starting with the learner's agenda about problems experienced and specific areas for improvement.

Whatever approach is used feedback should be:

- balanced and objective;
- descriptive, not judgmental;
- specific rather than general;
- focused on behaviour rather than personality;
- helpful and informative;
- checked out with the recipient;
- delivered in digestible amounts;
- solicited rather than imposed; and
- ideally focused only on things that can be changed.

Appraisal

Appraisal, a process that originated in the commercial sector, brings together formative assessment and feedback. It has been taken up in the professional world, including medicine and education, traditionally as part of a hierarchical system of performance review and career development. Many purposes of appraisal have been described, including:

- reinforcing acceptable and effective behaviour;
- identifying factors impairing performance;
- identifying educational and development needs, both individual and organizational;
- assessing how individuals can best contribute to achieving organizational aims;
- identifying situations where there is duplication of effort;
- developing a more collaborative style of management.

The process has been modified for use in non-hierarchical settings, as 'peer appraisal'. In general practice, this has been defined as:

a process in which GPs meet in pairs or groups to discuss and review their performance and activity in the practice, covering a wide range of topics.[28]

It can be undertaken in unidisciplinary and multidisciplinary settings, one-to-one or in a group. Although there is no standard format, it usually involves the following steps:

- review of past performance and achievements (strengths, weaknesses, and perceived needs);
- giving and receiving constructive feedback;
- agreeing goals and objectives.

It needs to be an on-going process, and documentation is required. There have been no systematic evaluations of peer appraisal, but there is some descriptive literature. For example, Jelley, in the North East of England, surveyed all practices in the region.[27] Although only a minority were involved in peer appraisal, several advantages and disadvantages were identified. It was felt to improve team cohesion and well-being, facilitate personal and professional development, promote reflection, and enable discussion of difficult topics in a safe environment. On the other hand, it was felt clear objectives may be difficult to set, conflicts between individual and practice needs were highlighted, it is time consuming and requires particular skills, and may become 'cosy' and non-challenging. A system of peer appraisal adopted in the USA and Australia, whereby a number of colleagues report on the performance of an individual, has proved reliable, and has been proposed as a possible approach for revalidation in the UK.[29]

Evaluation

Evaluation is literally attaching value to something. In educational terms it is a process of identifying and interpreting the effects and effectiveness of teaching and learning. Information is gathered about aspects of an educational event in order to make judgements about it. It should be a systematic process, implicit to which is the notion of change and development.[30,31]

There are many parallels with assessment, for example, evaluation often being added as a 'bolt-on' extra, with little thought given to its purpose and methods. In selecting appropriate indicators, the 'utility' equation described above has relevance, for example, in considering validity and reliability.

Broadly, there are four possible approaches:

• learner-oriented, predominantly focused on learner performance;
• programme-oriented, for example, related to intended learning outcomes;
• institution-oriented, often carried out by an external agency, for example the Quality Assurance Agency; and
• stakeholder-oriented, bearing in mind that evaluation inevitably has political implications.[31]

Kirkpatrick described four *levels* of evaluation, ranging from 'evaluation of reaction' ('How was it for you?'— much educational evaluation does not go beyond this) to 'evaluation of results', for example, changes in health outcomes.[32] Learners' perceptions of the value of an educational experience may change over time, thus timing of evaluation is an important consideration.

The outputs of evaluations are:

- evidence—i.e. the data;
- conclusions—the data given meaning through analysis and interpretation;
- judgements—values placed on the conclusions;
- recommendations—suggested courses of action.

Evaluation is not the same as research, not least because its findings are usually not generalizable, but demands similar methodological rigour if it is going to have any meaning. There are, however, some parallels with qualitative research. For example, because of the complexity of most educational situations, more than one method may be desirable in order to triangulate findings to increase their reliability.

Mentoring

Well established in other professions, mentoring is being increasingly adopted and adapted in primary care. The traditional model, whereby a senior person acts as guide and role model to a junior colleague, is being replaced by a less hierarchical approach consistent with the principles of adult learning. Co-tutoring, defined as 'a dialogue between two autonomous practitioners on a voluntary basis',[33] is a particular model of mentoring based on a peer relationship, which may enable professionals to enhance performance and handle stress more effectively. Evidence of its efficacy is beginning to emerge. Co-tutors meet regularly, giving each other time to talk through problems perceived to be obstructing personal or professional development. The agenda may cover both pastoral and educational issues. The process promotes insight and reflection, and enables change. There is obvious overlap with other educational approaches, for example, some models of appraisal or clinical supervision.

Whatever the model, the mentor may take on many roles: facilitator, counsellor, critical friend, information provider, role model, networker, companion on a journey, and coach. Key attributes of a mentor include listening and facilitating skills, being a respected person with sound job and organizational knowledge, ability to confront and challenge, a non-judgmental, empathic approach, and insight and tolerance.

Mentoring, increasingly recognized as an important potential component of CPD, will only become established if it receives institutional support, and is properly resourced, in terms of provision of protected time, and training and support for mentors.[34]

Groups, teams, and multiprofessional education

Effective primary care increasingly demands a group, or team approach. Indeed, much policy—for example, clinical governance and CPD—implicitly assumes health-care professionals will spend most of their time working and learning with others.

Learning in groups concords with many of the educational principles described thus far. It can be a powerful tool for achieving deep and enduring learning, building and maintaining a team, and achieving individual and organizational change. There is a large body of theory and understanding about groups and how they work most effectively.[35,36] Unfortunately, many people appear to be unaware of this, although most will recognize that inappropriate use of small group techniques can be at best ineffective, and at worst damaging both to individuals and the organization.

There are many definitions of a 'group', differing in emphasis and detail. However, it is generally agreed that members of a group have a common purpose, and that the interaction between them is different and more focused than casual or social encounters. Thus, a group shares an identity, a frame of reference, and common objectives. A team is a group in which, in addition, members generally divide labour and distribute functions.

There are a number of key issues to consider in respect of effective group functioning. Whereas *what* a group does will obviously vary from group to group, *how* it goes about it—the group process—generally follows a common pattern, involving purposeful activity, interaction, and a degree of reflection. Three dimensions of group behaviour have been described:

- *task* behaviour, focused on helping the group achieve its task;
- *group* behaviour, directed at helping the group survive and develop; and
- *individual* behaviour, focused on the needs of the individual.

Groups often have a natural life span and evolve and develop through several stages. The best known classification for group development was proposed by Tuckman, who described four stages:

- forming (when members first gather together);
- storming (when the rules and roles are disputed);
- norming (when rules and roles are agreed upon); and
- performing (when group eventually starts to work together).[37]

Failure to work through and resolve the (inevitable) conflicts of an earlier stage may result in problems later on.

Group size is an important issue, and the ideal group for effective and efficient function is said to be between five and eight members. Greater than this, and increasing effort has to be put into ensuring active participation and addressing individual needs, usually by breaking the larger group down into smaller units.

Working and learning in groups is particularly suited to activities such as complex tasks requiring input from several people, developing interpersonal skills or attitudes, group skills, including facilitation and leadership skills, developing and applying new ideas, and managing change. Groups have their limitations as well as strengths and, indeed, there are situations in which group work is inappropriate, such as simply imparting information or addressing simple routine tasks.

There are many determinants of group effectiveness, including characteristics of individual members (their individual goals, ambitions and personal 'baggage'), understanding of the task and of the group process, attributes of the group (including size, developmental stage, skill mix, and how effectively it is facilitated or led), the task (its nature, clarity of objectives, whether it is achievable), and the setting (including the physical environment, and time and resources available). One obvious factor is seating arrangements—it is amazing how often people fail to recognize the importance of being face to face in promoting interaction. The characteristics of an ideal group are shown in Box 5.2.

Box 5.2   Characteristics of an 'ideal group'

Members

- Work cooperatively, not in competition
- Get along with each other
- Receive incentives and rewards collectively, not individually
- Understand group processes

Group

- Between 5 and 8 members
- Autonomy to address the task
- Effective facilitation or leadership
- Adequate resources, and time to complete the task
- Operates in a supportive context

Task

- Involves all members, draws on skills of individuals, requires coordination
- Concrete, relevant and achievable
- Clear objectives, a beginning and an end, measurable indicators of success or outcome

---

There are three possible roles in a group: leader, facilitator, and member. Leading and facilitating require different skills. The leader usually has a vested interest in obtaining a particular outcome, and there is an expectation that he/she will direct the group process to that end. A facilitator's role, on the other hand, is to help the group meet its agreed objectives and overcome problems in the group process. A facilitator must take a broad view of the tasks and should remain as neutral as possible. This makes the task of being an *internal* facilitator (i.e. from within the group) quite difficult, even potentially damaging. A wide range of atttributes are required for effective facilitation, begging the need for training for the role. One of the facilitator's tasks is to help the group deal with any challenging behaviour of its members. Box 5.3 shows a classification of different types of difficult behaviour; strategies for dealing with them can be found in the literature on groups.[36]

Box 5.3   Challenging behaviours in groups

Members who talk too much

- The dominator
- The enthusiast
- The confuser

Members who talk inappropriately

- The digressor
- The debater
- The know-all
- The joker

Members who talk very little

- The timid or reticent
- The passive aggressor

Other forms of destructive behaviour

- The whinger
- The rank-puller
- The politician
- The neurotic

From Elwyn *et al.*[36]

Of course, it is possible that such behaviour may be a (healthy) sign that the group process itself needs addressing, and the facilitator should be attuned to this possibility. Another important task is maintaining participative safety and encouraging active participation. In a small, well-established group, this will occur naturally, but in a larger group it may be necessary to use one or more technique to promote interaction. Such techniques include:

- 'buzz groups'
- snowballing, or pyramids
- syndicate groups
- role play
- brainstorming.

Again, these are well described in the literature.[36]

Group work, which is assuming an increasingly important role in primary care, can be very creative and productive. However, it can also be frustrating and even damaging when things go wrong. Unfortunately, there are many reasons why groups become dysfunctional, such as members behaving inappropriately, poor facilitation, and the group becoming too comfortable and uncritical (displaying so-called 'group think').

Multiprofessional education

The organization, content and delivery of health and social care is becoming more complex, and the multiprofessional team is assuming an increasingly central role in the eyes of both policy makers and educators. It seems common sense that learning together should make *working* together more effective, efficient, and enjoyable. Shared learning goes under a number of different names: multiprofessional, interprofessional, interdisciplinary, multidisciplinary. Whatever the term used, the basic idea is the same, i.e. an opportunity for members of more than one health or social care profession to learn together. The benefits claimed for multiprofessional education (MPE) are simple but profound: increased collaboration between different professionals in their work, leading to better care and improved outcomes for patients. However, although studies of MPE in both the UK and elsewhere have demonstrated increases in mutual understanding and respect, improved communication and more positive attitudes, there is little published evidence that it actually promotes active collaboration, let alone more effective and efficient working, or improved patient outcomes.[38] The principles of effective MPE are shown in Box 5.4.[39]

Influences on the effectiveness of multiprofessional groups or teams have been described under three headings:[40]

- structural (e.g. organizational issues such as status, autonomy, rewards, practical constraints, lines of accountability);

Box 5.4   Principles of effective interprofessional education

- Works to improve the quality of care
- Focuses on the needs of, and involves service users and carers
- Promotes interprofessional collaboration
- Encourages professions to learn with, from, and about one another
- Enhances practice within professions
- Respects the integrity and contribution of each profession
- Increases professional satisfaction

From Barr and Waterton[39]

- cultural (e.g. different ideologies, value systems, and expectations);
- interpersonal (e.g. communication, group process).

Harden described three additional areas to be considered in organizing MPE:

- context (including the stage or phase of education, the setting, the topics, and the educational strategies);
- goals (MPE may have as it goals: common core competencies; development of a multiskilled workforce with breakdown of professional boundaries; mutual understanding of roles; and general skills which will facilitate teamworking);
- approach (a continuum of approaches ranging from professional isolation to 'trans-professional').

The task of facilitating a multiprofessional group, whether to help them work or learn together (or both!) is inevitably more challenging than a uniprofessional group. A range of factors, referred to above, related to organizational and cultural issues, may cause difficulty or dysfunction, and must be borne in mind. A problem-based or task-based approach may be particularly appropriate in the multiprofessional setting.

Significant event analysis

This is a group approach to case discussion proposed as an important tool for clinical governance.[41] It goes under a variety of names, including significant event audit, and critical event, or incident analysis, and has been shown to be an acceptable and effective method for team-based, multiprofessional audit in primary care.[42,43] It is a mechanism for exploring noteworthy events in practice, with the purpose of learning from, and celebrating good practice, as well as improving suboptimal practice. By reviewing individual cases in this way, the team can generate standards to improve the quality of care. Significant events can be clinical, administrative, or organizational. Ideally, all team members involved in the particular case participate in the discussion, describing and clarifying first what actually occurred, the subsequent events and issues raised, why the incident was perceived to represent either good or poor practice, and whether and what action is required. Records should be kept, including details of proposed actions (if any), and there are considerable benefits to 'revisiting' the case at a subsequent review discussion, thus giving the opportunity to 'close the loop'. The discussion will be more effective if facilitated, and there are strong arguments in favour of external facilitation.[42]

Portfolio-based learning and personal learning plans

Portfolio-based learning

This approach, derived from the graphic arts, has been taken up in other settings, including school education, nursing, and general practice. It involves collecting evidence that learning has taken place, but is based on more than a simple description of experience. It requires demonstration that some sort of transformation through reflection has taken place. Portfolios potentially have use in three areas:

- personal development, as a way of tracking progress;
- formative assessment; and
- summative assessment.

Although relatively little critical appraisal of the effectiveness and efficiency of portfolios has been published, their potential benefits are congruent with the principles of adult learning and reflective practice.[44,45]

Documentation can include:

- records of experiences or critical incidents;
- details of reading undertaken (e.g. journal articles or books);
- projects;
- formal educational sessions attended;
- videotaped consultations.

Evidence of learning comes through written reflection on each of these, discussing what has been learned, what is still to be learned, and plans for new learning.

Portfolios are neither a soft option, nor a 'quick fix'. They are highly personal documents (begging the need for ground rules, such as who has access to the portfolio, what should be documented, and so on). They focus on the *quality* not quantity of learning, and require a significant time commitment from both learner and appraiser. Their use is growing in health-care education and evidence of benefit is beginning to emerge. A major issue remains the problem of using them summatively. In terms of their 'utility' as an assessment instrument, there are problems, particularly with reliability, largely as a result of attempting to assess non-standardized material 'with methods that stem from a reductionist philosophy . . . trapped by our need to compare like with like'.[46]

Personal learning plans

The use of personal learning plans (PLPs) is similarly gaining ground in health-care education. Also known under several other names, such as learning contracts,

PLPs are a way of identifying and documenting what the learner needs to know and why, how they will go about learning it and in what time frame, how they will know when learning is complete, and links with past and future experience and learning. PLPs are thus fully congruent with principles of adult learning (Box 5.1). There is no set format for a PLP, but it should include details of educational needs, learning objectives or outcomes, strategies for achieving the outcomes and what resources may be needed, and a record of outcomes and progress.[47,48]

Personal and practice development plans, first introduced in proposals for CPD in general practice,[49] essentially bring together PLPs and the portfolio approach. Both approaches also tie in with appraisal and mentoring.

Understanding and managing change

There is a plethora of models and theories describing change and change management at all levels—organization, team, and individual. Many share key features, such as the need for clear objectives, committed leadership, fostering ownership and effective communication. Another common theme is the sequence of steps involved (often referred to as a cycle or spiral):

- What is the current situation?
- How could it be improved?
- How can this be achieved?
- How will we know when we get there?

However, one of the most crucial considerations is the importance of context. A model only has meaning when adapted to the context in which it is to be applied; what works in one setting may not work in another apparently similar setting because of subtle differences, for example, the local history of change, or relationships between key players. Different stakeholders—clinicians, managers, economists, politicians, educators, the public—may have very different ideas about the best strategies for change, often based as much on personal belief as on evidence.[50]

Whilst recognizing there is no perfect answer, one practical model originally described in relation to change in medical education, which is grounded in experience, rather than theory, provides a useful framework.[51] Core activities in the process, and associated key issues are shown in Table 5.1.

Table 5.1   A model of managing change in medical education

Core activity	Key issues
Establish the need for change	Need for communication; change as opportunity
Power to act	Ownership; stakeholders; borrowed power
Design the innovation	Feasibility; resources; barriers and success factors
Consult	Leadership; communication; teamwork; refinement
Publicize the change widely	Presentation; further refinement
Agree detailed plans	Clear objectives
Implement changes	Demonstration projects; strategy; stakeholders
Provide support	Overcome difficulties and smooth new pathways
Modify plans if necessary	Accept further refinements; compensate losers
Evaluate outcomes	Strategy; objectives met; benefits and costs

After Gale and Grant.[51]

It is also important for those involved in facilitating change to anticipate possible barriers, whether at the level of the institution (for example, lack of ownership, or poor leadership) or the individual (for example, lack of time or resources, misunderstanding of the change, or fear of the unknown).

At the level of day-to-day practice, key factors influencing the likelihood of a new idea being adopted include:[51]

- relative complexity;
- relative advantage over existing practice;
- opportunity to observe the innovation in use;
- compatibility with existing practice;
- opportunity to try the innovation.

Five categories of adopters of change have been described: innovators, early adopters, early majority, late adopters, and laggards. Each group has its characteristic features, values, and communication behaviour. The roles of the 'idea champion' and local opinion leaders have also been emphasized.[52]

Health professionals need to be able to manage continuing change, whether this is at the level of acquiring a new skill or implementing guidelines, or at the level of major organizational change, such as new working practices. In any case, education and professional development, and management of change are completely interwoven processes.

Challenges

The evidence in favour of adopting more learner-centred and strategic approaches to personal and practice development is overwhelming, and this is reflected in policy documents, both academic and political. However, a number of tensions will need to be acknowledged, and challenges embraced.

Education versus training

A distinction is often drawn between 'education' and 'training', the former implying a process of personal growth and development for the purpose of learning, the latter the acquisition of a set of skills for a specific job, with little critical reflection involved. However, the terms are often used interchangeably, and in any case it is something of a false dichotomy. It is hard to imagine an intelligent person learning a set of skills without putting them into a broader context. (Conversely, members of the public may appreciate an automatic, non-reflective response from a health professional if unfortunate enough to require cardiopulmonary resuscitation!) Nonetheless, the distinction serves to highlight wider tensions between 'education' and 'service'. The busy practitioner will often feel there is no time for lofty notions such as personal development and reflection, and this highlights the importance of trying to embed learning in everyday practice, and at a more strategic level, of developing partnerships between education and service.[53]

Adult learning versus performance management

Primary care is increasingly becoming a managed environment in which professional practice is guided and monitored by an increasing number of processes and systems, many of them new and, at the time of writing, untested. At least some of these processes are at variance with the principles of adult learning, and could result in conflict with potentially adverse effects, not least a damaging effect on morale. Nonetheless it does not make sense to separate CME and CPD from the overall management process, and in theory at least, a system such as clinical governance offers a framework within which some of these tensions can be reconciled.[54]

Closing the loop and following through

Whatever method of needs assessment, learning strategy or feedback process is used, the crucial question is whether the loop of learning is closed and followed through. Strategies needs to be in place to ensure that the cycle of learning continues feeding back into practice when required (which will probably be in almost every instance!) and that the processes and, where possible, outcomes are continually evaluated. It is important to ask not just 'What happened?', but also 'What happened next?'.[55]

The learning organization—rhetoric or reality?

In a 'learning organization' (a concept derived from the business world), learning is seen as the only sustainable competitive advantage one organization might have over another. In the words of one author, they are:

organisations where people continually expand their capacity to create the results they truly desire, where new and expansive patterns of thinking are nurtured, where collective aspiration is set free, and where people are continually learning to learn together.[56]

Learning organizations need to be adaptive to their external environment, continually enhance their capability to change and adapt, develop collective as well as individual learning, and use the results of learning to achieve a better product. Clearly such a philosophy concords with adult learning principles and recognizes the importance of the learning environment, and in a health-care setting is a context in which, for example, clinical governance could operate successfully. Indeed, the learning organization has been proposed as an aspiration for primary care at the level of both the practice and the primary care trust, indeed throughout the NHS[57,58] However, the (extensive) literature on the subject of 'learning organizations' is largely descriptive and as with many other management theories and models, there is little evidence in support of its efficacy and practicality. Furthermore, the philosophy is clearly at variance with the culture of regulation, monitoring and blame that at least *some* primary care professionals feel prevails. Health managers and educators alike would be well advised not to beat the learning organization 'drum' too loudly, particularly at a time of radical change such as the introduction of primary care trusts.

Summary

This chapter reviews key principles underpinning effective learning and change management relevant to the challenges facing general practice and primary care in the new NHS. They will obviously need to be put into an appropriate and enabling organizational context if they are to bear fruit.

References

1.   Harden RM, Grant J, Buckley G, Hart IR. BEME Guide No 1: best evidence medical education. *Medical Teacher* 1999; **21**: 553–62.
2.   Knowles MS. *The Adult Learner: a Neglected Species*. Houston: Gulf, 1990.

3. Kaufman DM, Mann KV, Jennett PA. *Teaching and Learning in Medical Education: how Theory can inform Practice*. Edinburgh: Association for the Study of Medical Education, 2000.

4. Chastonay P, Brenner E, Peel S, Guilbert J-J. The need for more efficacy and relevance in medical education. *Medical Education* 1996; **30**: 235–8.

5. Norman GR. The adult learner: a mythical species. *Academic Medicine* 1999; **74**: 886–9.

6. Grant J, Chambers E, Jackson G. *The Good CPD Guide*. Sutton : Reed Healthcare Publishing, 1999.

7. Eve R. Learning with PUNs and DENs—a method for determining educational needs and the evaluation of its use in primary care. *Education for General Practice* 2000; **11**: 73–9.

8. Kurtz S, Silverman J, Draper J. *Teaching and Learning Communication Skills in Medicine*. Oxford: Radcliffe Medical Press, 1998.

9. Maslow AH. *Motivation and Personality*. New York: Harper and Row, 1970.

10. Davis DA, Thomson MA, Oxman AD, Haynes RB. Evidence for the effectiveness of CME. A review of 50 randomized controlled trials. *Journal of the American Medical Association* 1992; **268**: 1111–17.

11. Oxman AD, Thomson MA, Davis DA, Haynes RB. No magic bullets: a systematic review of 102 trials of interventions to improve professional practice. *Canadian Medical Association Journal* 1995; **153**: 1423–31.

12. Honey P, Mumford A. *The Manual of Learning Styles*, 3rd edn. Maidenhead: P Honey, 1992.

13. Boud D, Feletti G, eds. *The Challenge of Problem-based Learning*. London: Kogan Page, 1991.

14. David T, Patel L, Burdett K, Rangachari P. *Problem-based Learning in Medicine*. London: The Royal Society of Medicine, 1999.

15. Norman GR, Schmidt HG. The psychological basis of problem-based learning: a review of the evidence. *Academic Medicine* 1992; **67**: 657–65.

16. Finucane PM, Johnson SM, Prideaux DJ. Problem-based learning: its rationale and efficacy. *Medical Journal of Australia* 1998; **168**: 445–8.

17. Downey P, O'Brien D. Problem-based learning in GP vocational training. *Education for General Practice* 1999; **10**: 265–71.

18. Sackett DL, Rosenberg WM, Gray JA, Haynes RB, Richardson WS. Evidence-based medicine: what it is and what it isn't. *British Medical Journal* 1996; **312**: 71–2.

19. Sackett DL, Richardson WS, Rosenberg W, Haynes RB. *Evidence-based Medicine. How to Practise and Teach EBM*. Edinburgh: Churchill Livingstone, 1997.

20. Stanton F, Grant J. Approaches to experiential learning, course delivery and validation in medicine. A background document. *Medical Education* 1999; **33**: 282–97.

21. Kolb DA. *Experiential learning: experience as the source of learning development*. Englewood Cliffs (NJ): Prentice Hall, 1984.

22. Al-Shehri A. Learning by reflection in general practice: a study report. *Education for General Practice* 1995; **7**: 237–48.

23. Harden RM, Laidlaw JM, Ker JS, Mitchell HE. Task-based learning: an educational strategy for undergraduate, postgraduate and continuing

medical education. *AMEE Education Guide No 7*. Dundee: Association for Medical Education in Europe, 1996.

24. Newble D, Jolly B, Wakeford R, eds. *The Certification and Recertification of Doctors. Issues in the Assessment of Clinical Competence*. Cambridge: Cambridge University Press, 1994.

25. Rolfe I, McPherson J. Formative assessment; how am I doing? *Lancet* 1995; **345**: 837–9.

26. Van der Vleuten CPM. The assessment of professional competence: developments, research and practical implications. *Advances in Health Sciences Education* 1996; **1**: 41–67.

27. Pendleton D, Schofield T, Tate P. *The Consultation: an Approach to Learning and Teaching*. Oxford: Oxford University Press, 1984.

28. Jelley D. *A Peer Appraisal Package*. Newcastle upon Tyne: Postgraduate Institute for Medicine and Dentistry, 2000.

29. Southgate L, Pringle M. Revalidation in the United Kingdom: general principles based on experience in general practice. *British Medical Journal* 1999; 319: 1180–3.

30. Pitts J, Percy D, Coles C. Evaluating teaching. *Education for General Practice* 1995; **6**: 13–18.

31. Wilkes M, Bligh J. Evaluating educational interventions. *British Medical Journal* 1999; **318**: 1269–72.

32. Hutchinson L. Evaluating and researching the effectiveness of educational interventions. *British Medical Journal* 1999; **318**: 1267–9.

33. Alliott R. Facilitatory mentoring in general practice. *British Medical Journal (Career Focus)* 1996; **Classified supplement 28 September**: 2–3.

34. Freeman R. *Mentoring in General Practice*. Oxford: Butterworth Heinemann, 1998.

35. Crosby J. Learning in small groups. AMEE Medical Education Guide No 8. *Medical Teacher* 1997; **19**: 189–202.

36. Elwyn G, Greenhalgh T, Macfarlane F. *Groups: a Guide to Small Group Work in Healthcare, Management, Education and Research*. Oxford: Radcliffe Medical Press, 2000.

37. Tuckman BW. Developmental sequence in small groups. *Psychological Bulletin* 1965; **63**: 384–99.

38. Zwarenstein M, Atkins J, Barr H, Hammick M, Koppel I, Reeves S. A systematic review of interprofessional education. *Journal of Interprofessional Care* 1999; **13**: 417–24.

39. Barr H, Waterton S. Summary of a CAIPE Survey: interprofessional education in health and social care in the United Kingdom. *Journal of Interprofessional Care* 1996; **10**: 297–303.

40. Harden RM. Effective multiprofessional education: a three-dimensional model. *Medical Teacher* 1998; **20**: 402–8.

41. Pringle M. Significant event auditing. In: Van Zwanenberg T, Harrison J, eds. *Clinical Governenace in Primary Care*. Oxford: Radcliffe Medical Press, 1999.

42. Robinson LA, Stacy R, Spencer JA, Bhopal RS. How to do it: use facilitated case discussions for significant event auditing. *British Medical Journal* 1995; **311**: 315–18.

43. Pringle M, Bradley C, Carmichael C, Wallis H, Moore A. *Significant Event Auditing. Occasional Paper No 70.* London: Royal College of General Practitioners, 1995.

44. Snadden D, Thomas M. The use of portfolio learning in medical education. *Medical Teacher* 1998; **20**: 192–9.

45. Challis M. Portfolio-based learning and assessment in medical education. AMEE Medical Education Guide No 11 (revised). *Medical Teacher* 1999; **21**: 370–86.

46. Snadden D. Portfolios—attempting to measure the unmeasurable? *Medical Education* 1999; **33**: 478–9.

47. Challis M. Personal learning plans. AMEE Medical Education Guide No 19. *Medical Teacher* 2000; **22**: 225–36.

48. Rughani A. *The GP's Guide to Personal Development Plans.* Oxford: Radcliffe Medical Press, 2000.

49. Chief Medical Officer. *Review of Continuing Professional Development in General Practice.* London: Department of Health, 1998.

50. Grol R. Beliefs and evidence in changing clinical practice. *British Medical Journal* 1997; **315**: 418–21.

51. Gale R, Grant JR. *Managing Change in a Medical Context: Guidelines for Action.* London: The Joint Centre, 1990.

52. Stocking B. Promoting change in clinical care. *Quality in Health Care* 1992; **1**: 56–60.

53. Gillam S, Eversley J, Snell J, Wallace P. *Building Bridges. The Future of GP Education—Developing Partnerships with the Service.* London: King's Fund, 1999.

54. Donaldson L. Clinical governance: a quality concept. In: van Zwanenberg T, Harrison J, eds. *Clinical Governance in Primary Care.* Oxford: Radcliffe Medical Press, 1999.

55. Eraut M. Do continuing professional development models promote one-dimensional thinking? *Medical Education* 2001; **35**: 8–11.

56. Senge P. *The Fifth Discipline: the Art and Practice of the Learning Organization.* New York: Doubleday, 1990.

57. Bhanot S, Percy D. Learning for general practitioners in the new NHS. *Education for General Practice* 1999; **10**: 225–32.

58. Davies HTO, Nutley SM. Developing learning organisations in the new NHS. *British Medical Journal* 2000; **320**: 998–1001.

Further reading

Adult learning, self-directed learning

Coles C. A review of learner-centred education and its applications in primary care. *Education for General Practice* 1994; **5**: 19–25.

Kaufman DM, Mann KV, Jennett PA. *Teaching and Learning in Medical Education: How Theory can inform Practice.* Edinburgh: ASME, 2000.

Needs assessment (including PUNs and DENs)

Grant J, Chambers E, Jackson G. *The Good CPD Guide.* Sutton: Reed Healthcare Publishing, 1999.
Rughani A. *The GP's Guide to Personal Development Plans.* Oxford: Radcliffe Medical Press, 2000.

Problem-based learning

David T, Patel L, Burdett K, Rangachari P. *Problem-based Learning in Medicine.* London: The Royal Society of Medicine, 1999.

Evidence-based practice

Sackett DL, Richardson WS, Rosenberg W, Haynes RB. *Evidence-based Medicine. How to Practise and Teach EBM.* Edinburgh: Churchill Livingstone, 1997.

Experiential learning, reflective practice

Al-Shehri A. Learning by reflection in general practice: a study report. *Education for General Practice* 1995; **7**: 237–48.
Stanton F, Grant J. Approaches to experiential learning, course delivery and validation in medicine. A background document. *Medical Education* 1999; **33**: 282–97.

Assessment

Jolly B, Grant J. *The Good Assessment Guide. A Practical Guide to Assessment and Appraisal for Higher Specialist Training.* London: Joint Centre for Education in Medicine, 1997.
Van der Vleuten CPM. The assessment of professional competence: developments, research and practical implications. *Advances in Health Sciences Education* 1996; **1**: 41–67.

Feedback

Kurtz S, Silverman J, Draper J. *Teaching and Learning Communication Skills in Medicine.* Oxford: Radcliffe Medical Press, 1998.
Pendleton D, Schofield T, Tate P. *The Consultation: an Approach to Learning and Teaching.* Oxford: Oxford University Press, 1984.

Appraisal

Jelley D. *A Peer Appraisal Package.* Newcastle upon Tyne: Postgraduate Institute for Medicine and Dentistry, 2000.
Haman H, Irvine S, Jelley D. *The peer appraisal hand book for general practitioners.* Oxford Medical Medical Press, 2001.

Evaluation

Coles CR, Grant JG. Curriculum evaluation in medical and health care education. *Medical Education* 1985; **19**: 405–22.
Pitts J, Percy D, Coles C. Evaluating teaching. *Education for General Practice* 1995; **6**: 13–18.

Mentoring

Freeman R. *Mentoring in General Practice.* Oxford: Butterworth-Heinemann, 1998.

Groups

Crosby J. Learning in small groups. AMEE Medical Education Guide No 8. *Medical Teacher* 1997; **19**: 189–202.
Elwyn G, Greenhalgh T, Macfarlane F. *Groups: a Guide to Small Group Work in Healthcare, Management, Education and Research.* Oxford: Radcliffe Medical Press, 2000.

Portfolio-based learning

Challis M. Portfolio-based learning and assessment in medical education. AMEE Medical Education Guide No 11 (revised). *Medical Teacher* 1999; **21**: 370–86.
Snadden D, Thomas M. The use of portfolio learning in medical education. *Medical Teacher* 1998; **20**: 192–9.

Personal learning plans

Challis M. AMEE Medical Education Guide No 19: Personal learning plans. *Medical Teacher* 2000; **22**: 225–36.
Rughani A. *The GP's Guide to Personal Development Plans.* Oxford: Radcliffe Medical Press, 2000.

Multiprofessional education

Harden RM. Effective multiprofessional education: a three-dimensional model. *Medical Teacher* 1998; **20**: 402–8.
Parsell G, Bligh J. Educational principles underpinning successful shared learning. *Medical Teacher* 1998; **20**: 522–9.

Significant event analysis

Pringle M, Bradley C, Carmichael C, Wallis H, Moore A. *Significant Event Auditing.* Occasional Paper No 70. London: Royal College of General Practitioners, 1995.
Robinson LA, Stacy R, Spencer JA, Bhopal RS. How to do it: use facilitated case discussions for significant event auditing. *British Medical Journal* 1995; **311**: 315–18.

Change management

Gale R, Grant JR. *Managing Change in a Medical Context: Guidelines for Action.* London: The Joint Centre, 1990.
Greenhalgh T. *British Journal of General Practice* 2000; **50**: 76–7, 164–5, 252–3, 340–1, 424–5, 514–15. A series of papers about change management.

6 The principles of assessment

REED BOWDEN AND NEIL JACKSON

The historical setting

It may come as a surprise to a young doctor entering general practice today to learn that well within living memory it was possible for a man—it was usually a man—to qualify as a doctor one day and start work in a practice the next day, alone and unsupervised. The only assessment beyond finals was the loyalty and affection, or otherwise, of his patients.

In 1950 pre-registration house jobs were introduced, but essentially the career path remained unobstructed by any formal assessment until mandatory training for general practitioners (GPs) began in 1979.

By that time the three great changes in practice over the last 50 years were well developed. More and more women were becoming GPs; there was a trend towards working in partnerships and multidisciplinary teams; and the need for continuing assessment was increasingly acknowledged. At the same time the perception of GPs within the profession (and more slowly among the general public) was changing.

When aspiring doctors of the 1940s and 1950s applied to medical school, there were always a few places for those following in their fathers' footsteps, or who were useful on the rugby field, and provided they were not too dullwitted they might be allowed in. This may have mattered little in a low-tech world where hard work and a comforting manner went a long way. As late as 1966 the eminent physician Lord Moran could say:

A medical career was a ladder on which those of outstanding merit rose to be consultants and others fell off to be [general] practitioners.[1]

These days most people recognize that the intellectual demands of practice are as great as those of any hospital speciality. Indeed, much that was previously seen as the work of hospital consultants is now routinely dealt with in general practice, with asthma and diabetes the obvious examples. But as we shall see, general practice has not yet found the courage to make its entry requirements as rigorous as medicine or surgery.

What is the point of assessment?

From the viewpoint of the general public, few would dispute that the main purpose of assessment is to provide reassurance that a practitioner is competent and remains competent. *Competence*, of course, means having the ability to do the job. It is an essential ingredient of *good performance*, which means actually doing the job well, but competence alone does not guarantee this. Performance needs separate assessment.

Assessment also helps in determining who has the competence to carry out particular clinical tasks, how many such people there are and where they are; it is therefore a valuable tool in *workforce planning*. It can have discriminatory powers, to rank people in order of competence and to *aid selection*. Assessment, including self-assessment, can motivate individuals to greater *self-development*. Lastly, assessment drives learning. It can therefore be used strategically to strengthen desirable learning behaviour. This effect can be used in *curriculum development*, for Vocational Training Schemes, for instance. Another example was provided when the Royal College of General Practitioners required its membership candidates to provide certificates of competence in cardiopulmonary resuscitation procedures.

A representation of some of these principles was given by Miller,[2] who expressed his idea as a pyramid of performance, with 'knows' as its base, then higher levels of 'knows how', 'shows how', and 'does'. The levels can be assessed by factual tests for 'knows', context-based tests for 'knows how', performance in simulated situations for 'shows how', and observation of real performance for 'does'.

How to become a GP

- Qualify
- Obtain Provisional Registration
- Complete Pre-Registration House Appointments satisfactorily
- Obtain Full Registration

What other assessments does our hypothetical new entrant face?

- Educationally approved Senior House Officer (SHO) posts
- A post with an Approved GP Trainer

After full registration, he (it is at least as likely to be she, but for brevity let us agree on he) will be required to undergo 3 more years of training. He may choose a 3-year vocational training scheme (VTS), with entry controlled by the deanery, which is the regional organization responsible for postgraduate medical education; or construct his own scheme by putting together a set of four educationally approved Senior House Officer (SHO) posts followed by a year as a GP registrar with an approved trainer, coordinated through the deanery. Satisfactory completion of each post is confirmed by the issue of a certificate, a VTR2 for each hospital post and a VTR1 for the practice attachment, VTR referring to the Vocational Training Regulations. Three hospital posts and 18 months with a practice is an approved variation. It will be appreciated that the regulations define the time to be spent in training, not the skills to be acquired. In other words, GP training is not fundamentally curriculum-based.

Some deaneries include a form of *gate-in test* with their entry interviews, particularly for entry to schemes (see later).

Summative Assessment

In order to obtain his VTR1, the new GP must pass a four-part Summative Assessment (SA) examination during his time as a registrar. This is described in detail later.

Submission for Membership of the Royal College (optional)

He may also choose to attempt the Membership of the Royal College of General Practitioners (MRCGP) during or shortly after the registrar year, to demonstrate ability above the basic level of SA.

Revalidation (pending)

As a principal, or indeed when working in any non-principal role in practice, there will soon be annual appraisals leading to a revalidation review every 5 years all the way through to retirement.

The European dimension

British vocational training regulations have had to work alongside the regulations of other nations of the European Community (EC) in order to satisfy freedom of movement and employment obligations. This has not always been accepted without demur, as some EC countries have been perceived as having less stringent GP training criteria. Amended legislation in the European parliament in June 2000 has gone some way to easing the situation, as the 3-year training period for GPs now applies across the community.

Assessments later in the GP's career

Older doctors, established in practice, may wish to become MRCGP by the standard route or by assessment of performance, or Fellows by assessment if they are already Members.

An increasing number of GPs are opting to work for higher degrees in general practice.

Revalidation assessments will be touched on later.

Doctors who struggle or underperform

Inevitably there will be some doctors whose performance does not remain at an acceptable level as their careers progress. There may be a number of reasons for this, often working in combination. They include the doctor's health, with burnout an ever-present danger, an adverse working environment, and failure to maintain an educational commitment. The particular challenges of dealing with these situations are covered in Chapter 4. The point to be made here is that many of the assessment and performance management methods described below can be used for this group also.

Before looking in more detail at assessment in general practice, let us consider the nature of educational assessments and the qualities they must have to be acceptable.

Formative and summative assessment

The defining feature of formative assessment (FA) is the intention to encourage a learner along an educational route towards an objective. If the objective is not achieved, further time and teaching are allowed so that the learner can try again, and so on. FA has the merit of being able to determine strengths and weaknesses, and to enable the logging and mapping of educational progress. Despite its name it can, alone, be used to build a comprehensive picture of educational achievement.

With summative assessment (SA) a snapshot of ability is taken at a defined moment, and if the required standard is not met the learner has failed and the process stops.

The reader will have spotted the paradox in these descriptions. For FA to be 100% formative, the learner should be granted an infinite number of attempts at the task; and for SA to be truly summative it should be a once-only experience without retakes. In reality there may come a time when, despite every encouragement, the learner has still not reached the objective that FA was meant to bring him to, whereas SA is rather like the driving test: you can take it again but you must not drive alone until you have been successful.

In summary, formative assessment:

- breaks up the learning pathway into manageable modules;
- allows repeated attempts to master the content of each module;
- is not perceived as threatening.

Summative assessment:

- is an end-point examination;
- can block intended career progression (a 'high stakes' examination);
- is perceived as threatening.

The qualities of assessment

Candidates expect their examinations to be *fair*. The assessment should reflect the curriculum they were asked to follow, and the curriculum should include all the knowledge and competencies, or at least all the core knowledge and competencies, that their intended career requires. Allied to fairness is the concept of *transparency*; in other words the mechanisms by which the examination is run, the marking schedules and appeal procedures are all laid bare. An examination which guards its processes from scrutiny may be perfectly fair, but transparency enhances the feeling that it really is.

Matching the assessment to the curriculum has two important and linked functions. It directs learning; it is a rare student who will spend time on parts of the curriculum that are not going to be assessed.[3] And it is what makes the assessment *valid*. Not only must it be valid, but the ideal assessment must reflect the examinees' ability accurately, be able to rank them in order of ability, and to show that the same rank-order still applies—give or take a few inevitable changes—if it is repeated. These are the qualities that make an assessment *reliable* and *discriminatory*. The discriminatory qualities of an assessment are broadly correlated with difficulty. Everybody knows the capital of France, quite a few people know the capital of Peru, but it is a rare citizen who knows the capital of Burkina Faso.

The more methods an examination uses to assess candidates the more reliable the examination becomes, provided each method is itself valid. The statisticians have a great deal to say about validity and reliability, but cleverness with numbers can sometimes tempt us to forget the basic design difficulties, particularly around the curriculum. What does a GP need to know? What does a GP really need to know? How much can be left to Continuing Medical Education (CME) later on, whether structured CME or the informal learning of simply doing the job? Can anyone, however wise, imagine what a GP's life will be like in 2020 or even 2010? The hard truth is that workforce planners have to try in order to achieve the best possible fit between the needs of health service provision and the interests and aspirations of the people who will fill the posts.

A further quality that an examination must have is that it should be *feasible*. In other words, the logistics of setting it up and running it must not be insurmountable. The final necessary quality is *legal defensibility*. There are two parts to this. There is the ability to defend the examination against a charge of unfairness from a candidate who has failed it; and the ability to defend it against the accusations of a patient who has suffered at the hands of a candidate who was declared competent by it. No examination can be perfect, but these considerations become crucial for processes such as SA, as failure in this will mean the intended career pathway is no longer open to that doctor. Such an effect demands that the whole process is as robust in an educational sense as it can possibly be.

In summary then, the hallmarks of the best examinations are:

- validity
- reliability
- maximizing reliability by using several assessment methods, all valid
- discriminatory ability
- transparency
- legal defensibility
- feasibility.

Gate-in assessments

The transfer of funds from the General Medical Services (GMS) budget to the Medical and Dental Educational Levy (MADEL) means that deaneries have now assumed responsibility for admitting doctors to GP registrar posts. A few deaneries have begun to insist on a test of some kind as part of the selection process. One method, from Wessex (F Smith, personal communication, 2000) is to include a questionnaire in the structured application form. There are two questions on communication skills and difficulties, another on psychological or social factors in management, one on motivation for entering general practice, and one on the personal skills the applicant believes they can offer.

In Sheffield (PW Lane, personal communication, 2000), the intention is for the selection process to include a test in the style of an Observed Structured Clinical Examination (OSCE), with several 'stations', covering group work, clinical scenarios, interviews, and written work.

The United Kingdom Committee of Regional Advisers' Summative Assessment Process

In order to enter unsupervised practice GP registrars have to pass a four-part assessment during their time at their training practice, which is usually 1 year. It may be extended at the discretion of the Dean (or Director) of Postgraduate General Practice Education (DPGPE) if any of the modules have to be retaken, or exceptionally for other reasons. The SA process is currently run by the deaneries on behalf of the United Kingdom Committee of Regional Advisers (UKCRA), who founded it as a professionally led process in the first instance. Their methodology was approved by the Joint Committee on Postgraduate Training for General Practice (JCPTGP). This body is the 'competent authority', charged by the government to oversee the whole process when it became law in 1997. It is likely, under the provisions of the National Health Service (NHS) Plan[4] that the JCPTGP will merge with the Specialist Training Authority to form a new Medical Education Standards Board.

The multiple choice questions (MCQs)

There are various types of MCQ examination. The one used in SA is perhaps the most familiar. A stem question is followed by a number of branch statements which candidates must rate as true or false, shading an area with pencil to indicate their choice. MCQ examinations began in the USA and their use has grown enormously over the last 40 years.[5] They have the advantage of sampling knowledge over a wide range of subjects in an acceptable time. Their forte is to assess factual knowledge; their principal drawback is that they only assess factual knowledge, and not problem-solving ability. To remedy this, the MCQs have been supplemented by Extended Matching Questions (EMQs), in which the candidate is given a list of possible diagnoses, followed by a number of clinical scenarios. For each scenario, they must choose the likeliest diagnosis from the list.[6]

The written submission

By the time SA became mandatory, progressive practices had already accepted the need to audit their processes and outcomes in order to improve patient services and push ahead with quality initiatives. SA played its part in this trend by requiring GP registrars to produce an audit.[7] It was accepted at first that a year did not allow enough time to revisit the subject of the audit to demonstrate change. Soon, however, this 'closing of the audit cycle' will become a requirement, not unreasonably, as computerization is now universal in training practices, and this makes data retrieval much simpler.[8]

Some educationalists, while admitting the importance of audit, felt that registrars should be given the scope to produce other forms of written submission if they wished, including family studies, significant event analysis, and so on. It proved difficult to produce a marking schedule for such a range of possible submissions, but eventually the Yorkshire deanery devised one which has obtained approval from the JCPTGP.[9,10] For the moment, however, most GP registrars continue to submit an audit, and to pass this module they must choose a subject which has clear potential for improving patient benefit or the efficient running of the practice, and to relate it to previous work on the subject, quoting references if available. The methodology must be sound, and there should be evidence of teamwork in choosing and investigating the audit subject and applying the lessons learned. A few relevant references and an exposition of how the practice should change completes the project, and (from 2001) registrars will be encouraged to revisit the subject to demonstrate change, if any.

The written submission is a part of the process which can be done during the hospital SHO jobs, although the subject must be relevant to general practice.

The demonstration of consulting skills

Until the beginning of 2000, consulting skills had to be assessed by a videotape of the registrar consulting with patients. From that date, however, an alternative method, the Simulated Surgery, became available. Each method has its advantages and disadvantages.

Videotaped consultations

Every video is different from every other, and all videos contain a mixed bag of consultations, though regulations require a range of problems to be presented on the tape, of varying difficulty, in order to demonstrate the registrar's range of ability. In other respects, the regulations are not prescriptive concerning what is presented. Registrars generally edit their tapes, very sensibly, as everyone is entitled to present themselves to their best advantage, and the editing and rejection process is a formative learning experience in its own right. Videos are accompanied by a logbook in which the registrar has the chance to demonstrate understanding of the process of the consultation, to add extra information, which may help the assessor make an accurate judgement, and to show that any minor shortcomings on the tape have been noted as a learning opportunity. Logbooks may of course have a fictional element to them, which the assessors can only guess at. Videos can strain the assessors' indulgence by their technical shortcomings; it can be difficult to provide good sound and picture, with the patient and doctor shown well enough to pick up facial and other non-verbal cues, and quite impossible when there is a group consultation such as a mother with two or three children. All in all, it is no surprise to find that making the video can take up several weeks for some registrars, and can engender high levels of anxiety. The Simulated Surgery, described later, is already showing signs of becoming a preferred alternative, but it is likely that video will continue to be chosen by many because of the accommodation that has been reached between the SA process and the MRCGP examination. The College brought in its video module in the autumn of 1996, partly to answer the criticism that their examination contained no direct observation of doctors at work. From spring 2001 videos sent in by practice registrars for MRCGP purposes will count as SA passes if they are College passes. If they fail at College level they will be returned by the College to deaneries to go through the SA assessment system.

Simulated Surgery

Simulated Surgery has a number of advantages over video, and some disadvantages of its own. The 'patients' that the registrars will meet are modelled closely on real consultations, which the doctors who suggested them felt were representative of practice, or which stretched their own consulting skills. The mixture of consultations is under the control of the organizers, and each cohort of examinees sees the same group of patients. Marking can be done by the actors playing the patients or by an observer. A disadvantage is that it is impossible to simulate certain types of patient. A young child cannot be simulated except by presenting the problem vicariously via a parent or other adult. Both methods, video and simulation, are open to the criticism that doctors may not perform in the same way when unobserved as they do under examination conditions. There is evidence, however, that those who know how to consult well do consult well, observed and unobserved. One research method, which has been used in this area, is the 'masked patient'. In this method, the doctor agrees with the researcher that over a specified period the researcher may send along a number of undercover patients to assess the doctor's work directly. The evidence is that such patients are almost never identified by the doctor, and that the correlation with observed skills is good.[11]

The Structured Trainer's Report

This final part of SA is a booklet in which the trainer or a suitably skilled colleague keeps a record of the registrar's observed ability in a range of competencies. It covers a number of practical procedures, some extremely basic, and matters of organization and self-discipline such as the use of time and the ability to identify strengths and weaknesses in his or her own performance. It has the incidental advantage that its contents and preamble form a useful basis for the trainer and registrar to map out a curriculum for the year.

Many young doctors choose to enter themselves for the MRCGP examination, either in their registrar year or shortly afterwards. In particular, many will wish to attempt the video module while they are still registrars as the equipment may not be readily available when they move on to work elsewhere. The College has never striven to be exclusive or elitist, but its membership examination is calibrated to demonstrate a degree of ability beyond that of SA. There is a cumulative pass rate of between 75 and 80% of those attempting it. General practice is unique among medical specialities in not demanding membership of its college as a requirement for its fully fledged independent practitioners, a fact that justifies the earlier statement that we have not had the courage to insist on the highest standard for entry. The reader may speculate on the possible reasons for this. Among them it is fair to include the political embarrassment of having, for a few years at least, a group of qualified doctors who are unlicensed to work independently anywhere within the profession, and who may be regarded as less visible in general practice than elsewhere.

Quality and governance: the educational consequences

Most of us may still claim medicine as an art, but it is an art that sends deep roots into science. In order to offer the highest quality service to our patients we are obliged to look to the science for guidance on best practice. Clinical governance (see Chapter 4) is a quality assurance framework which includes that obligation along with others, such as learning from mistakes and keeping ourselves up to date by well-chosen continuing medical education. The young GP who has recently been successful in SA and possibly the membership has a starting point for continuous learning and should have developed an appetite for it; the established doctor may find it harder to learn what it is he needs to learn. Identifying learning needs forms part of the personal development plans which will soon be required of us. Doctors in practice are also required to submit practice professional development plans, which include plans for team learning, audit, and much else. The whole subject has been given a keener edge with the announcement that all doctors will be subject to annual appraisals which were scheduled to begin in 2001, leading to a 5-yearly revalidation on which the right to continue in practice will depend. The content of the revalidation package is not yet definite in every detail, but we know it will include a requirement to show that self-assessed learning needs have been addressed.

Self-assessment of learning needs

The temptation is to attend to the areas where we sense a deficiency, or to areas we find interesting. We may also try to define our educational needs by *reflection*, perhaps by keeping a *reflective diary* of practice. The difficulty is that these subjective methods may not lead us to the areas of greatest learning need. More objective methods are required as well, and such methods are available.

PUNs and DENs

This method, developed by Eve,[12] depends on keeping a record of consultations where the doctor, having done his best, is nevertheless left with a perception that the patient has not received all that might have been offered (a patient's unmet need, or PUN). When PUNs are found to cluster in a particular subject area, the doctor has identified a DEN (a doctor's educational need), which can then be addressed. This method seems so simple it may feel like cheating, but it is a powerful and effective indicator of where the educational needs are.

Books and CD-ROMs

There are many MCQ and EMQ question-books available, mostly designed for revision for the MRCGP, but well-suited to on-going self-assessment as well.[13] Some journals, including one of the free newspapers, regularly publish MCQ tests.[14] For those who prefer an electronic alternative, various teaching CDs exist. A helpful example, covering a wide range of GP work, are the PEP-CDs put out by the Scottish Council of the RCGP.

Other methods

Other methods to guide learning include *critical event analysis*, in which the doctors and other involved team members examine events such as unexpected deaths, new diagnoses of malignancy, and other important matters. A practice's *complaints* process may also suggest learning needs.

A stable partnership in which the no-blame culture is well established may allow the *doctors to suggest learning topics to each other*.

Mentoring

Mentoring is a technique that touches on assessment though without the hard statistical edge. The essence of it is the seeking out, by a doctor who feels the need for sympathetic advice and help, of an experienced colleague who is prepared to give sustained and non-judgemental advice based on a frank analysis of the seeker's professional situation and the mentor's experience. A doctor's mentor would usually be an older doctor, though it is not necessary for the mentor to be either older or a doctor. Mentoring is confidential by its very nature and therefore it is difficult to offer an objective analysis of it. An exposition of this important subject is given by Freeman in Chapter 14, and in her book.[15]

Assessing the educational needs of the whole team

For many primary health-care teams, the central feature of team-member evaluation is *appraisal*. Regular, usually annual appraisal should be a feature of the working life of all members of the primary health-care team (PHCT). The essence of an appraisal is that protected time is set aside for each person to meet with their appraiser to review their work. The job description may be corrected and updated, and the successes and difficulties of the past year are talked through. Pay and conditions are usually dealt with on a separate occasion. The career path and aspirations are at the heart of the appraisal, and the educational requirements to achieve these ambitions are agreed. It is likely that each team member will find one or more organizations that offer education tailored to their needs. AMSPAR (the Association of Medical Secretaries, Practice Managers, Administrators and Receptionists), for example, supports practice managers and office staff, and nurses can look to the English National Board, which approves university-accredited courses which can build towards a degree, or to special courses such as the Stratford asthma course, which provide certificates of satisfactory attendance for the nurse's educational portfolio. There may be a regional organization (such as EQUIP, the Education and Quality in Practice organization in Essex) running courses for all categories of primary care workers.

The appraisers are usually senior people doing the same kind of work as the person appraised. When it comes to appraising the doctors themselves, the situation can become a little more difficult. Many doctors have conveniently ignored appraisal. Others have found co-appraising each other works well, and yet others see their own appraisal as being an appropriate task for the practice manager. For doctors, all these systems are likely to be swept aside when revalidation begins, to be replaced by appraisal by an experienced local colleague who is not a partner. There is more about appraisal in Chapter 5.

The strengths and weaknesses of learning in groups and teams across professional boundaries are expounded in Chapter 3.

Patient expectations

Patients, like other users of services, are increasingly likely to demand the highest quality that can be delivered. They are entitled to assume that new doctors have been properly assessed and that systems are in place to ensure that they and their PHCT colleagues remain competent and up to date. The government, which is in effect the employer of most doctors in Britain, not only has the right to know that its staff are of the highest calibre, but also the duty to provide the time and the means to allow them to achieve that status. Doctors themselves have a professional duty to maintain their knowledge and skills. Nevertheless, humans and the systems they construct are fallible. Mishaps will continue to occur and some patients will suffer harm. Our immediate response when this happens should be to look first at the structures and systems in which the harm occurred. We know that health-care workers strive to do their best; only occasionally will there be an unequivocal lapse by an individual.[16,17]

Assessment and learning in bigger units

All practices are required to direct their work by the principles of clinical governance, which have already been mentioned. Primary care groups and trusts (PCGs and PCTs) have begun to respond by instituting health improvement plans and by producing disease management protocols and guidelines on prescribing. They are ideally placed to become learning environments and providers of education of all types. Some have already chosen to hold study days for their entire membership, when service provision is covered by emergency arrangements for a few hours while all their practices study together. In some regions, PCGs have benefited by having GP tutors (now often called primary care tutors) appointed to work directly with them.[18]

Assessment and the nation's primary care needs

These are difficult days for British primary care. There is a shortage of doctors and nurses, which cannot be corrected for some years. We have a promise of more money every year for 5 years, with annual increments sufficient to increase NHS funding by one-third in real terms over that time.[4] There is no definite indication of how much will come to primary care.

The perennial argument over how much national ill-health can be ascribed to poverty and other social disadvantages and should be tackled outside the health service is as loud as ever.

There is disagreement over which parts of primary care should be provided by doctors, and which can be delivered by nurse practitioners and prescribers, by the NHS Direct telephone advice service, walk-in centres, pharmacists, and not least by patients themselves by way of increased over-the-counter availability.

Assessment methods will bear on all these questions. Where there is evidence for best practice, it must be heeded. We will have to assess who has the competencies to provide what we require, are there enough of them and are they where the need is greatest? Above all, we will need assessment, both self-assessment and external assessment, to allow primary care professionals to address their educational needs against a backdrop of relentless change.

References

1. Wolstenholme G, ed. *Lives of the Fellows of the Royal College of Physicians. Munk's Roll.* Oxford: IRL Press, 1984; **7**: 409.

2.   Miller GE. The assessment of clinical skills/competence/performance. *Academic Medicine (Supplement)* 1990; **65**: S63–7.
3.   Newble D, Jaeger K.: The effect of assessment and examinations on the learning of medical students. *Medical Education* 1983; **17**: 165–71.
4.   Department of Health. *The NHS Plan*. London: The Stationery Office, 2000.
5.   Case SM, Swanson DB. *Constructing Written Test Questions for the Basic and Clinical Sciences*, 2nd edn. Philadelphia, PA: National Board of Medical Examiners, 1998.
6.   Case SM, Swanson DB. Extended matching items: a practical alternative to free-response questions. *Teaching and Learning in Medicine* 1993; **5**(2): 107–15.
7.   Lough JRM, McKay J, Murray TS. Audit and summative assessment: a criterion-referenced marking schedule. *British Journal of General Practice* 1995; **45**: 607–9.
8.   Lough JRM, Murray TS. Audit and summative assessment: a completed audit cycle. *Medical Education* 2001; 35(4): 357–63.
9.   Evans AJ, Singleton C, Nolan PJ, Hall WW. Summative assessment of general practice registrars' projects; deciding on criteria and developing a marking schedule. *Education for General Practice* 1996; **7**: 229–36.
10. Evans AJ, Nolan PJ, Bogle S, Hall WW, Bahrami J. Summative assessment of general practice registrars' projects; reliability of the Yorkshire schedule. *Education for General Practice* 1997; **8**: 40–7.
11. Rethans JJ, Sturmans F, Drop R, van der Vleuten C. Assessment of the performance of general practitioners by the use of standardized (simulated) patients. *British Journal of General Practice* 1991; **41**(344): 97–9.
12. Eve R. Learning with PUNs and DENs—a method for determining educational needs and the evaluation of its use in primary care. *Education for General Practice* 2000; **11**: 73–9.
13. Ellis & Elliott, *MRCGP Practice Papers: MCQs and EMQs*, 2nd edn. Pastest 1999.
14. Moulds A. 'Doctor' newspaper, passim. The Moulds items appear weekly in free " Doctor " newspaper, page number variable. Published by Reed Healthcare Publishing.
15. Freeman R. *Mentoring in General Practice*. Oxford: Butterworth-Heinemann, 1998.
16. Berwick DM, Leape LL. Reducing errors in medicine. *British Medical Journal* 1999; **318**: 136–7.
17. Leape LL. and Berwick DM.(editorial). Safe healthcare: are we up to it? British Medical Journal 2000; **320**: 725–727.
18. Burton J, Jackson NR, McEwen Y. GP tutors work-based learning and primary care groups. *Education for General Practice* 1999; **10**: 417–22.

7 Quality, audit, and education and training

JOHN SCHOFIELD AND
NEIL JACKSON

Introduction

Our hope is to convince you that there is merit in considering quality methods in the development of primary care educational programmes. The significance of these ideas not only encompasses the education and training of medical staff but also the provision for the 'customer' of the best of services and the permeating of a quality culture throughout the health care environment.

Some understanding of the principles and methods of quality systems will allow us to relate their application, now and in the future, to educational structures. Wherever possible, reference to papers and texts on the subject are attached together with the Internet sites, which today are such an important source of information and reference.

The political atmosphere is very pro-quality in health care at the present time. Not only is this reflected in the medical profession by publications,[1] conferences[2] and research centres,[3] but by the promotion of quality thinking in government papers.[4] The same ideas are now established internationally, giving us a breadth and depth of models to consider.

As there is some variance as to how terms are used, we have included a brief list of definitions at the end of the chapter.

Background and philosophy

The ideas of quality can be condensed into three kernels of
wisdom:

- focus on the needs of the 'customer';
- evolutionary change and improvement;
- a culture of mutual support and blame avoidance.

Historically, quality ideas started to come together in the
1920s and 1930s in the USA. There was at that time a
huge shift towards the manufacture of complex goods for
the consumer. It became apparent that a new philosophy
was needed to organize such vast systems. The simplest of
ideas, proposed by Shewhart,[5] was to plan what you were
going to do first, then do it, and have some way of checking what you had done. In other words he developed a
feedback loop (Figure 7.1). The result of this method is an
incremental shift in the quality of the service.

Checking or auditing a system can be very difficult and
it was here that the next big improvement was made by
the application of basic statistical methods. Deming[6] developed ways of looking at the whole system and it was he
who identified four interlocking features for successful
organizations:

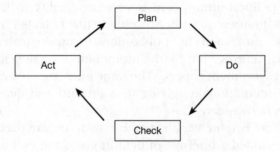

Figure 7.1 The feedback loop.

- an understanding of systems;
- an understanding of a theory of knowledge;
- an understanding of variation;
- an understanding of psychology and human behaviour.

The last aspect, the understanding of human behaviour and motivation, has proved the most significant of all in the development of quality cultures. Of particular interest here is the work of Belbin[7] of the organization of groups.

The Japanese, who enthusiastically embraced quality after the war, have also been very interested in how the group can bring about change in a much more effective way than the individual. Taiichi Ohno of Toyota is of particular interest and a description of his work can be found in the book by Yasuhiro Monden.[8]

The success of the application of these principles in industry has opened the question as to whether they are equally applicable to service industries such as health care. The person who has done more than anyone to develop this idea is Don Berwick in the USA.[9]

The economic case for quality

It is blindingly apparent to anyone working in health care anywhere in the world, be it the NHS in the UK, or the HMOs in the US, or any of the systems in Europe, that the pressure to contain costs is increasing. There are two alternatives to this problem: either the services that can be offered are rationed or better ways of working are found.

It has been the experience in industry that quality offers the possibility of delivering an improving service at a lower price. One only has to look at a modern television and compare it with one 20 years ago to realize the change.

We are not pretending that there is the possibility of this speed or degree of improvement in medical education, but it is worth considering whether some of the lessons learned in industry can be applied.

It is thought to cost something in the region of a quarter of a million pounds to turn a student into a general practitioner. To fail a student at the end of the process is both hugely expensive and emotionally draining for all concerned.

GPs make decisions on budget allocation of possibly a million pounds per year. When they are found to make a mistake the settlement costs can be very substantial, with amounts running into millions of pounds. This is reflected in the Medical Defence Union (MDU) subscription, which was £6 in 1970, but in 2000 is £2740 and increasing exponentially. The American figures for medical indemnity are of the order of 10 times those of the UK. Even these figures do not really represent the true cost to patients of medical negligence.

Only recently has the UK government decided to set up a system of recording mistakes or near mistakes (the National Clinical Incident Reporting System), which should allow for the identification of lacunae in the medical education system. It has been apparent from the MDU reports[10] and the cases coming before the General Medical Council (GMC)[11] that the same sorts of disasters happen again and again. This is by no means peculiar to the UK as there is extensive reporting of similar problems in the USA.[12]

A quality tool that is readily applicable here is a Pareto analysis. For the reader who wishes to look further into Pareto there are excellent web sites.[13] The key thing is that 80% of mistakes are caused by only 20% of causes. These can be analysed as a Pareto graph (Figure 7.2).

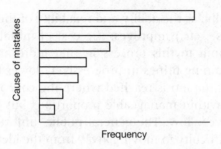

Figure 7.2   A Pareto graph.

The other classical area of cost saving is 'reworking'. What used to happen on a car production line was that as the vehicle was assembled the workers would have difficulty in certain areas, say getting the doors to fit properly, so the easiest way of coping was to pass the car on down the line and leave it to be sorted out later. The end result, as many readers will remember, was that the customer had to try and sort it out at the local garage. The cost is enormous both in trying to correct the defect and in the loss of confidence in the brand. (It will be interesting to see if we develop 'brands' in medical training not only from the medical school but in the postgraduate education field!)

The 'reworking' of doctors occurs with both the need to extend the training of those that have not passed their summative assessment and by the identification and support of 'poorly performing doctors'.

Finally, there is the concept of 'loss to society'; that is, if the health care supplied has not been of the best available, then the patient, the patient's family, the society, etc., have borne a loss compared with the optimal case. We are talking about an idealized state, which never exists, but the nearer you are able to get to it the more the society benefits. This is based on the work of Taguchi.[14]

Theoretically, as the ability and reliability of the worker (doctor, nurse, etc.) improves, the cost of mistakes falls. There is a limit to this process in that more and more expensive training brings in progressively lower benefits. An optimal situation is reached where the cost of education is kept within manageable proportions but the mistake rate is very low. The general public, unfortunately, have great difficulty in moving away from the idea of zero failure.

There are thus many possibilities for considerable cost savings to be made, which if ploughed back into well-structured quality educational systems could at the very least cover any increased costs and potentially would allow an expansion in the level of care available.

Systems of medical education

This is the really boring stuff: flow charts, procedures, log books, appraisals, control charts, feedback meetings, etc. It is like keeping the sewers cleaned out: very mucky and not very glamorous.

There is, first of all, the strategic thinking about how the system is currently working. Writing this down is by far the most important step. Looking at the system at present might appear as shown in Figure 7.3.

Next comes the auditing and feedback loops, which point the way to improvement. Incidentally, as quality is all about stealing good ideas from others and improving upon them; good practice, seen elsewhere, should be copied!

Mapping and logging is an important part of this process. Students must have a clear idea of where they are going and how that objective is to be measured. Frequent

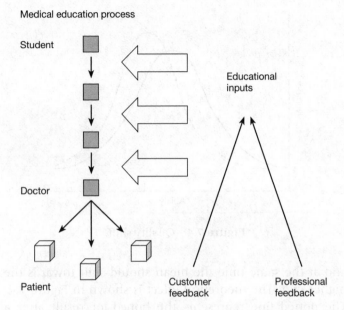

Figure 7.3 An example of the current system.

small reviews are the key to success, so that areas of work that are not clearly understood can be identified at the earliest opportunity and remedial action taken. As with the car production line, in the extreme case the whole education process needs to be stopped until the problem has been sorted out.

Assessment, appraisal, audit, call it what you will, is a must with quality systems. Going back to Dr Deming, without an understanding and access to data, you are lost. You cannot see what is happening and where you need to go to solve the problem. What we are trying to do is make sure that everyone has a good training without the possibility of a doctor having large or important gaps in knowledge or skills. Thus a graph of the distribution of abilities should move to less spread (smaller standard deviation)

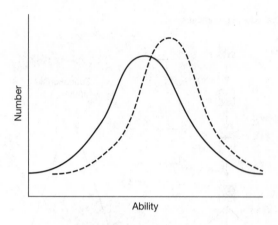

Figure 7.4   Quality shift.

and at the same time the mean should shift towards the higher end. The theoretical effect is shown in Figure 7.4. The dotted line represents the hoped-for result after a period of improvement.

With a systematic method it also becomes easier to differentiate between the failings of the educational process and the inability of the student to cope with the requirements. The latter situation should show up at the tail end of the ability distribution and the student can then be counselled to look for a less demanding career.

From a 'systems thinking' aspect, education can be thought of as an amplifier of effort. An efficient amplifier has both a positive and a negative feedback loop, which need to be in balance to produce the optimal outcome. There is a tendency to forget the positive encouragement of learners, which can have the effect of risk avoidance.

A clear understanding of not only what you are doing but also why you are doing it enables the systems to respond rapidly to changing demands.

Quality assurance and quality control

Internationally, there are methods of controlling the quality of products and services using set structures such as ISO 9000.[15] These have been extended to practices and similar ideas have been incorporated in the Royal College of General Practice 'Quality Practice Award'.

The importance of accrediting a person or an organization is that it offers to the customer the reassurance that the service they will receive is of a certain standard. It is extremely difficult for individuals to assess the quality of the medical service that they are receiving.

The other great problem in this area is the definition of the customer. Is this the patient at a particular point in their life when they are ill or is it the community, which might fear an epidemic, or is it the funding authority, be it the NHS or a Health-care management organization (HMO). The ideal quality system relies on identifying the customer and then trying to deliver the service that is sought.

The attempts to involve the public on a large scale have not been very inspiring. For instance, the Oregon study[16] produced results that would be difficult to justify from an ethical point of view.

There have been some studies from the Consumer Association looking at what patients want and these are interesting.[17] In particular, they point to communication skills as a key area that is valued. The current favourite method is to use 'focus groups' where people with differing perspectives are brought together to consider a subject. The various methods are nicely brought together by Ruth Chambers.[18]

If you are able to identify areas that are wanted, then these form the basis of measuring the success of what you are doing. Quality assurance (QA) is about putting in place educational structures that deliver a good service to the public. Each element is vital to the overall result and as elements are added, a QA system checks that the student or doctor has not only absorbed the ideas but is able to apply them.

If we then take the case of communication skills, we need literature that supports the best method of understanding these skills, methods that allow them to be taught, and checks, along the way, that the skill is being used successfully. In this case there is extensive research and literature on the consultation.[19] This can be incorporated in educational experiences both as a lecture and as actor-run simulations. The results can then be checked by simulated surgeries, OSCEs or video. Note that the desired result drives the whole process and not the final test.

The great advantage of QA is that everything is explicit, that is, you write down what you are planning to do, you do it, and then you have a checking method to make sure, very quickly, that it has been accomplished to the required standard. This may sound expensive and time consuming, but the final result is assured, that is, it comes consistently and reliably up to the customer's expectation. In the long run this offers the chance to reduce costly and preventable mistakes.

On the cost front, by increasing QA in the system the need for end-point testing 'quality control' (QC) is reduced. QC has traditionally been very important in medical education. The final examination and higher professional examinations were used as a check on the abilities of the doctor. These have the disadvantage of being able to measure only a part of the student's knowledge and skills. They have, however, an important use if QA methods have been adopted in giving a measure of the quality of the training programme of an organization. It is of interest that the most successful country in the US examination for foreign medical graduates, a QC system, is Australia, where QA systems have been widely used.[20]

Audit—an educational and assessment tool

It takes a lot of personal self-confidence and the support of colleagues to be able to audit one's work in medicine. Audit can be painful, especially when the consequences of mistakes are so enormous. In a confrontational atmosphere one can understand the reluctance of health workers to probe too deeply into problems or mistakes. Things are steadily moving on, and the recognition that the causes of problems are diffuse and complex has allowed a team approach to come to the fore.

Audit is now well established both in the education of all levels of medical education and in the long-term assessment of the quality of doctors' work. There are strong outside pressures to bring audit into regular use particularly with the introduction of clinical governance[21] and with the very public examples of failure reflected in the advice from the GMC.[22]

As an educational tool, it is ideal, as well-constructed audits allow a reflective aspect to one's work, and the opportunity to have team input and group decisions, resulting in the development of agreed working procedures. In assessment, the ability to present an audit for the summative assessment test at the end of GP training is now a requirement. Much work has been put into this by Murray Lough in the west of Scotland.[23] To those of us working in primary care education, it will be interesting to see if the efforts made to teach audit method will result in a generation of GPs who will use this skill in their everyday work.

When things go wrong

They always have and they always will!

This is about understanding people and systems. With the best will in the world, someone is sure to give the wrong injection or get the diagnosis wrong. In the same way, with the best efforts of the educators, the doctors whom they help to produce are not going to be perfect. One major difference between using quality in industry and in medical education is the variability of the raw material. We do not find a consistent basic student nor would we want to. The breadth and diversity of experience brings great strength to medicine. This is an interactive process where the teacher and the student are both interacting and moving forward.

When disasters do happen, the process should be to look at the whole system and try to understand where changes can be made and lessons learned. Our whole culture and legal system is diametrically against this, always trying to find scapegoats. A useful method of looking at problems is to use an Ishikawa[24] chart (Figure 7.5) to understand the

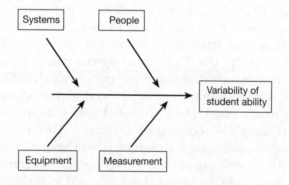

Figure 7.5   An Ishikawa chart, the basic structure.

possible reasons for failure. The idea is to brainstorm the problem using Pareto analysis to understand in a highly complex organization where problems are arising. It can be very easy to blame the tutors involved without consideration of the other aspects such as lack of basic equipment or training facilities.

The problems involved with trying to apportion blame are that no one will cooperate, it becomes impossible to identify areas for change and almost certainly the same thing will go wrong again.

Application in primary care

The customer has always liked good quality primary care when it has been available. This really reflects the need for personal continuing relationships, easy access, and relevant medicine. The funding bodies are also coming to appreciate this aspect of the health-care system. It is relatively cheap, effective, and popular.

Medical schools are increasingly moving towards patient-centred and problem-based learning (PBL).[25] This, together with systematic education programmes and regular assessment, are very much in line with quality ideas. The introduction to the patient's view of their problem is an example of the new way of thinking.

Having qualified, the doctor is now moving into a structured training programme. For general practice training in the UK there has been the introduction of the summative assessment at the end of the vocational training. We are only now getting round to documenting and recording what education is undertaken during the hospital training posts and we are far from making regular assessment and appraisal. Without clear systems, it will be impossible to look back and reflect on where improvements can be made. A must has to be the log book[26] as a first step. Two excellent books in the area of university education are *Managing Quality and Standards* by Colleen Liston[27] and *Teaching for Quality Learning at University* by John Biggs.[28]

With Continuing Medical Education (CME), the emphasis is moving to the Personal Development Plan (PDP) and the Practice Professional Development Plan (PPDP). Both these concepts have very strong resonance in quality theory. They rely on the plan, do, check, act system of steady improvement. The PPDP is particularly interesting as it is a move away from the traditional view of the doctor being responsible alone, to a team approach where progress is seen as the involvement and business of the whole practice. These have also allowed the acceptance of Lifelong Learning with associated Professional Revalidation.[29]

Richard Eve has developed a useful tool to assist in this reflective method, called PUNs (patients' unmet needs) and DENs (doctors' educational needs).[30]

Future challenges

The future is unpredictable as is very obvious once you look back on past predictions. There are, however, a few trends that have already started and will almost certainly persist for the near future:

- The computing power of your PC will continue to grow very fast.[31]
- Biotechnology will open up vast new possibilities.
- The cost of health care will grow faster than the price of a new Mercedes.
- Communication bandwidth will expand so that 'knowledge' is available to anyone, anytime, anywhere.[32]

- We are all getting older and will need more health care.
- People will still want a friend to talk to.

How does quality fit into this rapidly changing world?

The big challenge is not with the technology but with the communication skills of the people using it. We have recently seen the rejection of genetically modified foods by the general public and the questioning of medical advances in stem cell therapy.

What will be needed is medical staff able to understand and interpret the new opportunities and translate those into a form which is acceptable to the everyday patient. This has two elements: first, new ways of recognizing what the customer wants; and second, having structures that can rapidly respond to changing environments.

One of the great advances at Toyota was the idea of 'just in time' (JIT), that is, the production line was not covered in boxes of parts waiting to be assembled but items were ordered when the system showed that they were needed. This concept can now be extended to education in the form of 'just in time training' (JITT), where the development of a new health programme identifies educational need and this can be delivered to staff just ahead of requirement. Nice examples of this are the humanoid models now available for teaching such skills as 'keyhole surgery' and cardiac examination. The development of the Internet clearly has a function here. Most colleges now have sites, which support their training programmes and provide material for students to work on both before and after their course.

Computer use has now become practically ubiquitous in medicine and has the capability to deliver any information to the GP's desk instantaneously. That same information will also be available to the patient. What consequence does this have on medical education and assessment?

It seems that the old examination based on factual recall is of only limited use. First of all, the 'facts' seem to change, and second, the customer is just as able to access the latest knowledge as the expert, so will put little value on this facility. What is needed is the ability to sift out the best evidence available, understand the needs and wants of the patient, and communicate possible solutions.

A role for quality in primary care training

There seems little doubt that quality ideas will become established and developed in this field. The main driving forces are political and financial, which are constantly looking for ways of providing more and more reliable health care to the public without the need to raise taxes.

If applied well, quality ideas do have humane and positive aspects. There is the psychological leap towards blame avoidance, the concept of evolutionary change, allowing people to use and expand their existing skills, and the very real possibility that the wishes of the patient in communication skills can be addressed.

It is our hope that we have, if only briefly, presented this subject for further consideration. There are very real problems in applying quality, but we feel that it has much to offer.

Definitions

Audit   A method of measuring the quality of a service.
Benchmarking   A level to which one aims being the best in the field.

Criterion A measurable and meaningful marker of the quality of a service.

Feedback The concept by which changes in output are used to influence either in a positive or negative way the inputs to a system.

Just in time training (JITT) A system by which the need for and the provision of training is geared to the development of health-care programmes.

Procedure A clearly laid out method usually as a flow chart as to how to carry out a task, e.g. register a new patient.

Quality assurance (QA) A method by which the whole of the inputs of a process are organized to reduce the risk of the failure of the final service.

Quality Control (QC) A method of checking the final service to make sure that it passes the minimum standard.

Reworking The process by which a faulty product is corrected at the end of the normal production.

Standards A level to which one hopes to reach for a particular criterion.

System An overall entity that defines an area of activity. A system may well consist of a number of processes that interact in complex ways.

References

1   *Quality in Health Care*. London: BMJ Publishing Group. http://www. qualityhealthcare.com.
2. European Forum on Quality Improvement in Health Care. http:// www.quality.bmjpg.com.
3. The Institute for Healthcare Improvement. http://www.ihi.org.
4. The Secretary of State for Health. *A First Class Service, Quality in the New NHS*. London: Department of Health, 1998. http://www.open.gov.uk/ doh/newnhs/quality.html.
5. Shewhart WA. *Economic Control of Quality of Manufactured Product*. London: Macmillan, 1931.

6.   Deming WE. *Out of Crisis*. Boston, MA: Massachusetts Institute of Technology, 1982.
7.   Belbin RM. *Management Teams*. Oxford: Butterworth-Heinemann, 1981.
8.   Monden Y. *Toyota Production System*. London: Chapman & Hall, 1983.
9.   Berwick DM, Godfrey AB, Roessner J. *Curing Health Care, New Strategies for Quality Improvement*. San Francisco, CA: Jossey-Bass, 1990.
10. Norwell N. *The Journal of the MDU* 1999; **15**(2). http://www.themdu.com.
11. The GMC News Section. http://www.gmc-uk.org/standard/news/news.html.
12. Berwick DM. Reducing errors in medicine. *British Medical Journal* 1999; **319**: 136–7.
13. http://www.ecom.unimelb.edu.au/ecowww/rdixon/pareto.html.
14. http://mijuno.larc.nasa.gov/dfc/tm.html.
15. Taylor D. Quality and professionalism in health care: a review of current initiatives in the NHS. *British Medical Journal* 1996; **312**: 626–9.
16. *Oregon Consumer Scorecard Project*. US department of Health and Human Services, 1996.
17. GPs your verdict. *Which* 1992; **April**: 202–5.
18. Chambers R. *Involving Patients and the Public—How to do it better*. Oxford: Radcliffe Press, 2000.
19. Silverman J, Kurtz S, Draper J. *Skills for Communicating with Patients*. Oxford: Radcliffe Medical Press, 1998.
20. Winward ML. Performance of foreign medical graduates on the clinical science component of the US medical licensing examination. *The 8th International Ottawa Conference on Medical Education and Assessment*, 1998.
21. The Secretary of State for Health. *The New NHS. Modern. Dependable*. London: The Stationery Office, 1997.
22. The General Medical Council. *Maintaining Good Medical Practice*. London: GMC, 1998.
23. Lough JR, Murray TS. Teaching audit—lessons from summative assessment. *British Journal of General Practice* 1997; **47**: 829–30.
24. Ishikawa K. *Guide to Quality Control*. Asian Productivity Organization, 1976.
25. Neufeld VR, Woodward CA, MacLeod SM. The McMaster MD programme: a case study of renewal in medical education. *Acad Med* 1989; **64**: 423–32.
26. Paice E, Aitken M, Cowan G, Heard S. Trainee satisfaction before and after the Calman reforms of specialist training. *British Medical Journal* 2000; **320**: 832–6.
27. Liston C. *Managing Quality and Standards*. Milton Keynes: Open University Press, 1999.
28. Biggs J. *Teaching for Quality Learning at University*. Milton Keynes: Open University Press, 1999.
29. Regulation Policy Section. *Revalidating Doctors, Ensuring Standards, Securing the Future*. London: General Medical Council, 2000. http://www.gmc-uk.org.
30. Eve R. *PUNs and DENs*. eve97@msn.com.

31. The new economy, untangling economics. *The Economist* 2000; September 23.
32. The future of wireless WEB. *Scientific American* 2000; October.

8 Research methods in medical education

COMFORT OSONNAYA AND
YVONNE CARTER

Innovation in medical education is a global issue. Increasing needs and pressures from both within and outside medical institutions are obliging them to devote a great deal of efforts to improving and adapting their curricula and teaching methods.[1]

These factors include the desire to improve courses despite the ever-increasing body of knowledge, the changing role of the doctor in the community, and the recognition of the potential of postgraduate and continuing education as an integral component of professional training. One response to these pressures has been an increased interest in research in medical education.

Research is best conceived as the process of arriving at dependable solutions to problems through the planned and systematic collection, analysis, and interpretation of data. It is the most important tool for advancing knowledge, for promoting progress, and for enabling people to relate more effectively to their environment, to accomplish their purposes, and to resolve his conflicts.[2] When we use the term educational research, we likewise have in mind the application of the same principles to the problems of teaching and learning within the formal educational framework and to the clarification of issues having direct or indirect bearing on these concepts. The particular value of scientific research in education is that it will enable educators to develop the kind of sound knowledge base that characterizes other professions and disciplines; and one that will ensure education, a maturity and sense of progression.

The process of research is made up of a number of stages that the researcher must proceed through for the research project to be completed satisfactorily. The stages are outlined in Box 8.1.

The purpose of this chapter is to introduce the reader to the major·features of the research process. The type of information that informs decisions about how to undertake a research project is described and supported by examples from educational perspectives. The chapter is intended for use by educators in the health-care sector with little or no previous research knowledge or training. Readers who already have a basic knowledge of the research process may find the chapter useful for revision. Hence the aims of this chapter are to:

- explore how educational research ideas start;
- introduce the reader to different types of educational research;

Box 8.1   The research process

- Identifying the research problem
- Reviewing the literature
- Defining the methodology
- Ethical considerations
- Pilot study
- Data collection
- Data analysis and results
- Drawing conclusions, identifying limitations, dissemination and application of results leading to further research

---

- explain the basics of medical educational research methodology;
- identify the first steps in designing a feasible educational research project.

Identifying the research problem

Every research project starts with an idea. People come across situations in their daily lives about which they would like to know more, or understand better. People also wonder about phenomena that they come across and ask themselves questions like:

- Why has a particular thing happened?
- How could they stop this from happening?
- Does it happen anywhere else?

People review their performance and wonder how they can improve it by asking questions like:

- How can we do this better?
- Can we do this more quickly/cost-effectively/differently?
- Are people satisfied with our performance?

Turning these questions into a *researchable* idea is the first stage of the research process. Sometimes our original idea is too difficult to research because it would take too long to find out the answer or it would take too many resources. If this is the case, the original idea has to be narrowed down to a manageable focus. For example, we may want to know if we are doing a good job. This sounds reasonable. But whom do we ask in order to find out? And how do we define what is meant by 'a good job'? If we allow our students to submit work late they may think we're doing a marvellous job, but our managers might not be very happy if we are not assessing the work in time or delaying the teaching, learning, and assessment processes.

Although it has been widely accepted that identifying a researchable idea is basically the first stage of the research process, it is quite common for the idea to be modified as the researcher starts to plan the subsequent stages of the research process. The second stage of the process is reviewing the literature to clarify whether the idea needs to be researched or whether the answers to our questions already exist. The third stage of the research process is defining the methodology to be used in conducting the investigation. At this stage it may become clear that the research focus is still too big to be manageable or that the people who would be needed to provide the information cannot be easily accessed.

It is always a good idea, at an early stage, to try and identify a phrase that describes the focus of the research. The research idea or research problem as it is often described, can be stated as an aim, a question, or a hypothesis. Indeed, it may take more than one aim, question, or hypothesis to adequately describe the purpose of the intended research.

It is not the case that one type of research statement is better than another, but that some types of research are better described by using one rather than another method. Research which is concerned with exploring or describing phenomena often uses aims or research questions to describe the research problem, whereas research concerned with testing out an idea frequently uses a hypothesis.

The important element common to any research problem is that it should be researchable and able to be investigated. For example, the question 'what is a good teacher?' is not answerable because there is no single answer; different people and different groups would have varying ideas about what makes a good teacher. However, if the study sets out to investigate 'students' perceptions of what they see as a good teacher', this is researchable because students' perceptions can be investigated. The following rules should be observed in stating the research problem:[3,4]

- an aim must be achievable;
- a question must be answerable;
- a hypothesis must be testable.

Box 8.2   An example of a research problem

It is frequently possible to describe a research problem by using an aim, a question, or a hypothesis. For example, if we wanted to look at the types of curriculum problems most frequently seen in medical education settings, we could state this as:

Aim

The aim of the research is to identify the curriculum problems most frequently encountered in medical education.

Question

What curriculum problems are most frequently encountered in medical education?

Hypothesis

Curriculum development and evaluation issues are encountered more frequently than any other curriculum problems in medical education.

Reviewing the literature

As identified in the previous section, every research project starts with an idea, something which the researcher is interested in knowing more about or is worried about—something that is felt to be a problem or a knowledge gap that needs to be filled, but at the outset is often vague or too broad to be covered in one research project. More information is needed by the researcher in order for the problem to be refined to make it manageable and researchable. This is assisted by an appraisal of existing literature. Before embarking on any research project, the researcher should search and appraise existing literature. The literature review has several purposes as it provides answers to the following questions:

- What is currently known about the topic or issue?
- What aspects of the topic lack sufficient information?
- Are there any gaps?
- What research or investigation has previously been done in that area?
- What recommendations for further investigation have been previously made but not acted upon?
- What methods have previous researchers used to investigate the topic and were some methods better suited to the topic than others?

Completion of the literature review enables the researcher to revisit the original research idea and define the exact focus of the research problem. It has been stated that the literature review should put the research problem into context. A good literature review contains up-to-date details of the literature and a balanced review of differing viewpoints or findings. Reviewing the literature is not simply a case of identifying previous research: it involves critical review of the advantages and disadvantages of the research. In writing up the results of a literature search the researcher should present a logical coherent case for pursuing the study.

Detailed information on how to search and review the literature has been described on numerous occasions.[4,5]

Defining the methodology

Medical educators debate heatedly about which models of scientific research should be applied to the problems in academic medicine.[6] This dialogue is fuelled by conflicting loyalties to different paradigms of science, medicine, and education.

Once the researcher has decided on the focus of the project, the next stage is to develop a plan of investigation. In developing the plan, the researcher takes into consideration such things as:[7]

• What am I trying to find out?
• What sort of information do I need?
• What is the best way to collect the information?
• Where can I get the information from?
• How many people will I need to ask?
• How will I analyse and make sense of the information I collect?

Research in medical education can be defined in terms of the type of activities that take place. Hence, the term 'methodology' refers to all these matters regarding the structure and design of the research study. It deals with such issues as:

• the type of information required;

- the research design;
- the method of collecting data;
- the source of information—this is known as the 'sample'.

Quantitative versus qualitative research

The type of information required depends on the original research idea. If the researcher wants to collect measurable information about a topic this is referred to as 'quantitative research'. It looks at:

- how big the problem is;
- how many people are affected by it;
- how often something occurs;
- whether one thing is more or less important than another;
- whether some things occur more often than others.

The specific elements that the researcher tries to measure are called 'variables' and outcomes that the researcher is trying to establish are also variables—for example, degree of success, examination pass rate, levels of course improvement, and student satisfaction. Variables are also the features that may have an effect on the outcomes, for example a student's age, IQ, or academic status.

Some situations cannot be easily broken down into a set of variables. The best example is human behaviour: why students act the way they do or how they feel in certain circumstances. If the researcher is trying to understand something in more detail or to describe a situation so that people can understand it better, this is often better achieved through qualitative research. In qualitative research, attention is focused on answering questions such as:

- Why?

- In what way?
- What are the implications?

This is in contrast to asking: 'How many? How often?' How much? as occurs in quantitative research. Further features of quantitative and qualitative research are listed in Table 8.1.

The research design

After deciding on the type of data required, qualitative or quantitative, the next methodological decision to be taken is on the type of research that will best address the research problem. There are many different types of educational research designs. The choice of design depends on the research problem. Research can be carried out using experiments, correlational studies, surveys, case studies, action research, phenomenology, triangulation, historical research, *ex post facto* research, role playing, and interviews.

Experimental designs

Experiments are controlled investigations that try to establish cause and effect between two or more variables with the purpose of predicting outcomes, for example, whether one type of educational method is more effective than another in teaching a particular medical topic. There are several different kinds of experimental design, but the classic experimental design involves two groups—an intervention group and a control group. Information relevant to the research problem is collected on the subjects (people) in both groups. Then one group, the intervention group, receives some kind of special or different tuition (the intervention) whilst the control groups receives no tuition or the usual teaching. Information is then collected from both groups and analysed to see whether the outcomes of the

Table 8.1   Characteristics of quantitative and qualitative
research question methods

Quantitative	Qualitative
The emphasis is on collecting measurable information	Information can only be loosely measured: can be identified but not specifically measured
Data can be analysed statistically	Data cannot be statistically analysed
Data can be quickly collected so large samples can be used	Data collection is more time-consuming so uses smaller samples
Data can be collected from a distance so it can be collected from widely dispersed members of the population	Data are usually collected face to face, so collecting data from a widely dispersed sample is time-consuming and expensive—local samples tend to be used
Data collection tools are highly structured and are time-consuming to develop	Data collection tools are more loosely structured
Once the tool is developed, data collection is relatively quick and cheap to collect and analyse	Data collection and data analysis are time-consuming and comparatively expensive
The main forms of data collection are: questionnaire surveys, highly structured observation schedules and analysis of records.	The main forms of data collection are individual interviews, focus groups and less-structured observation

Adapted from Hancock.[3]

two groups are different or the same. Experiments are carried out by collecting quantitative data that are subjected to statistical tests, which assess the probability that the variables are linked in a cause-and-effect relationship. The essential feature of experimental research is that investigators deliberately control and manipulate the condition, which determine the events in which they are investigating.

Triangulation

Triangulation may be defined as the use of two or more methods of data collection in the study of some aspects of human behaviour. It is a technique of research to which many subscribe in principle, but which only a minority use in practice. The use of multiple methods, or the multi-method approach as it is sometimes called, contrasts with the ubiquitous but generally more vulnerable single-method approach that characterizes so much of research in the social sciences. By analogy, triangular techniques in the social sciences and education attempt to map out, or explain more fully, the richness or complexity of human behaviour by studying it from more than one standpoint and, in so doing, by making use of both quantitative and qualitative data.

The principle of triangulation is illustrated at its simplest in a typical attitude scale. If you examine the example in Box 8.3, you will find ten items making up an attitude scale measuring a teacher's view of his/her role. One item, or 'locational marker', by itself will tell us very little about a teacher's attitude in this respect.

However, ten such related, or 'vocational markers' will give a much fuller picture. Imagine now a detailed study of a class of students in a medical school, which involves teachers' ratings of students, school records, psychometric data, sociometric data, case studies, questionnaires, and

---

Box 8.3   A teacher's attitude to his/her role

The scale below measures the extent to which a teacher interprets his/her role in either 'educational' or 'academic' terms. In using different 'vocational markers', it gives a more representative picture of the respondent's orientation to his/her role and in so doing illustrates the principle of triangulation in simple form.

- A teacher should teach informally most of the time.
- A teacher should be emotionally involved with his/her students.
- A teacher should use many and varied materials.
- He/she should regard scholarly attitudes to be of primary importance for his students.
- He/she should develop most of the work done in class from the students' own interests.
- A teacher should get to know students as individuals.
- A teacher should use harsh reprimanding methods.
- A teacher should look out for students with serious personal problems.
- A teacher should maintain discipline at all times.
- A teacher should get his/her chief satisfaction from interest in his subject or from administrative work in the school, rather than from classroom teaching.

Source: adapted from Cohen and Mannion[7]

---

observation. Add to this the findings of investigations of similar classes in ten other medical schools and we then have an illustration of the principle of triangulation at a more complex level.

In its use of multiple methods, triangulation may utilize either normative or interpretative techniques or it may draw on methods from both these approaches and use them in combination (see Box 8.4).

Box 8.4 The principal types of triangulation used in research

Time triangulation

This type attempts to take into consideration the factors of change and process by utilizing cross-sectional and longitudinal designs.

Space triangulation

This type attempts to overcome the parochialism of studies conducted in the same country or within the same subculture by making use of cross-cultural techniques.

Combined levels of triangulation

This type uses more than one level of analysis from the three principal levels used in the social sciences, namely, the individual level, the interactive level (groups), and the level of collectivities (organizational, cultural, or societal).

Theoretical triangulation

This type draws upon alternative or competing theories in preference to utilizing one viewpoint only.

Investigator triangulation

This type engages more than one observer.

Methodological triangulation

This type uses either
- the same method on different occasions, or
- different methods on the same object of study.

Correlation studies

Like experimental designs, correlation studies also investigate the likelihood of a relationship between two variables but they are interested in identifying associations rather than cause and effect. For example, is there a relationship between a special student group and the number of teaching hours? A correlation study might find that students from a certain special group are more likely than students from other special groups to be allocated specialist teachers for certain kinds of academic problems. A correlation study does not prove that the student is having special tuition because he/she is from a particular special group. The findings are limited to demonstrating that there is an association. This means that students from that group are more likely to have specialist teachers. Correlation studies collect quantitative data, which are subjected to statistical tests that calculate the strength of the link of the correlation.

The ability of partial correlational techniques to clarify the strength and direction of associations between variables is demonstrated in a study by Halpin *et al.*[8] In an exploration of teachers' perceptions of the effects of in-service education, the authors report correlations between teaching (T), organization and policy (OP), attitudes and knowledge (AK), and the dependent variable, student attainment (SA).

The strength of these associations is shown in Box 8.5, suggesting that there is a strong tendency ($r = 0.68$) for teachers who claim a higher level of 'INSET effect' on the teaching dimension to claim also a higher level of effect on pupil attainment and *vice versa*. The correlations between both the dimensions OP and AK and SA, however, are much weaker ($r = 0.27$ and $r = 0.23$, respectively).

Box 8.5   Correlations between pupil attainments and teaching, organizations and policy, and attitudes and knowledge

Student attainment (SA)

Teaching (T): 0.68
Organization and oolicy (OP): 0.27
Attitudes and knowledge (AK): 0.23
n= 196

Adapted from Halpin *et al.*[8]

Halpin *et al.* investigates the relationships further by means of partial correlational techniques. Table 8.2 shows the association between various dimensions of effect and student attainment. The partial correlation between T and SA is calculated.

Case studies

Unlike the experimenter who manipulates variables to determine their causal significance or the surveyor who asks standardized questions of large, representative samples of individuals, the case study researcher typically

Table 8.2 Partial correlation between student attainment and teaching organization and policy, and attitude and knowledge

Correlates	Controlling for	Partial r
SA and T	OP and AK	0.66
SA and QP	T	0.14
SA and AK	T	0.09
		=196

Adapted from Halpin *et al.*[8]

observes the characteristics of an individual unit—a student, a class, a college, or a community. The purpose of such observation is to probe deeply and to analyse intensively the multifarious phenomena that constitute the life cycle of the unit with a view to establishing generalizations about the wider population to which that unit belongs.

Present antipathy towards the statistical-experimental paradigm has created something of a boom industry in case study research. Problematic students, dropouts, and substance-abusers, to say nothing of studies of all types of college, attest to the wide use of the case study in contemporary social science and educational research.[4] Such wide use is marked by an equally diverse range to techniques employed in the collection and analysis of both qualitative and quantitative data. Some of the advantages of a case study are provided in Box 8.6.

The case study is capable of serving multiple audiences. It reduces the dependence of the reader upon unstated implicit assumptions and makes the research process itself accessible. Case studies, therefore, may contribute towards the 'democratization' of decision making (and knowledge itself. At its best, they allow readers to judge the implications of a study for themselves.

Surveys

The survey is perhaps the most commonly used descriptive method in educational research. Typically, surveys gather data at a particular point in time with the intention of describing the nature of existing conditions, or identifying standards against which existing conditions can be compared, or determining the relationships that exist between specific events. Thus, surveys may vary in their levels of complexity from those, which provide simple frequency counts to those which present relational analysis.

Box 8.6   Possible advantages of case study

Case studies have a number of advantages that make them attractive to educational evaluators or researchers. Thus:

- Case study data, paradoxically, is 'strong in reality' but difficult to organize. By contrast, other research data is often 'weak in reality' but susceptible to ready organization.
- Case studies allow generalizations either about an instance or from an instance to a class. Their peculiar strength lies in their attention to the subtlety and complexity of the case in its own right.
- By carefully attending to social situations, case studies can represent something of the discrepancies or conflicts between the viewpoints held by participants.
- Case studies, considered as products, may form an archive of descriptive material sufficiently rich to admit subsequent reinterpretation.
- Case studies are 'a step to action' as they begin in a world of action and contribute to it.
- Case studies present research or evaluation data in a more publicly accessible form than other kinds of research report, although this virtue is to some extent bought at the *expense of their length*.

Surveys may be further differentiated in terms of their scope. A study of contemporary developments in medical education, for example, might encompass the whole of Europe; a study of subject choice, on the other hand, might be confined to one medical school.

Whether the survey is large scale and undertaken by some governmental bureau or small scale and carried out

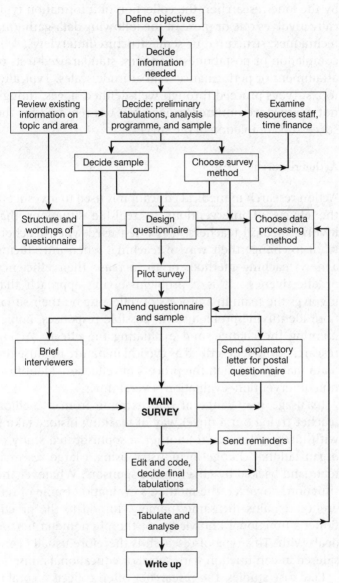

Figure 8.1 An example of various stages of a survey.
Adapted from Osonnaya and Osonnaya[4]

by the lone researcher, the collection of information typically involves one or more of the following data-gathering techniques: structured or semi-structuredinterviews, self-completion or postal questionnaires, standardized tests of attainment or performance, and attitude scales. Typically, too, surveys proceed through well-defined stages, though not every stage outlined in Figure 8.1 is required for the successful completion of the survey.

Action research

Action research in medical education is used to investigate the effects of interventions in real-life situations that involve medical teachers. It is often used when teachers want to change their way of teaching, when introducing a new teaching method, or to increase their efficiency or effectiveness. It is a problem-solving approach that involves the team in a process of reflecting on their situation, identifying problems and possible responses, implementing the change, and evaluating the effects. Action research is often described as cyclical in nature because the team may go through the process of reflection–identification–intervention–evaluation several times.

Its usage may range at one extreme from a medical teacher trying out a novel way of teaching history taking with his/her class to, at another, a sophisticated study of organizational change in industry using a large research team and backed by government sponsors. Whatever the situation, however, the method's evaluation frame of reference remains the same, namely, to add to the practitioner's functional knowledge of the phenomena he/she deals with. This type of research is therefore usually considered in conjunction with social or educational aims.

Like case studies, the researcher often collects a combination of qualitative and quantitative data.

Box 8.7 **The purposes of action research in education fall broadly into five categories**

- It is a means of remedying problems diagnosed in specific situations, or of improving in some way a given set of circumstances.

- It is a means of in-service training, thereby equipping teachers with new skills and methods, sharpening their analytical powers, and heightening their self-awareness.

- It is a means of injecting additional or innovatory approaches to teaching and learning into an on-going system which normally inhibits innovation and change.

- It is a means of improving the normally poor communications between the practising teacher and the academic researcher, and of remedying the failure of traditional research to give clear prescriptions.

- Although lacking the rigour of true scientific research, it is a means of providing a preferable alternative to the more subjective, impressionistic approach to problem solving in the classroom.

Phenomenology

Phenomenology literally means the study of phenomena. It is a way of describing elements that are part of the world in which we live: events, situations, experiences or concepts.[3] Phenomenological research investigates individuals' lived experience of events. It asks questions like: 'what does it mean to the individual to be involved in this situation, what effect does it have on that individual's life, their feelings, and their behaviour?' One example of phenomenological research would be an investigation into the experience of teaching a student with dyslexia. The study would consider the meaning of teaching in that context, the components of teaching and the impact—negative and positive—it has on teachers' lives.

Historical research

Historical research has been defined as the systematic and objective location, evaluation, and synthesis of evidence in order to establish facts and draw conclusions about past events.

Historical research in education can also show how and why educational theories and practices developed. The values of historical research in education are outlined in Box 8.8. It enables educators to use former practices to evaluate newer, emerging ones. Recurrent trends can be more easily identified and assessed from an historical standpoint; witness, for example, the various guises in

---

Box 8.8   The values of historical research in education

The values of historical research can been categorized as follows:

- it enables solutions to contemporary problems to be sought in the past;
- it throws light on present and future trends;
- it stresses the relative importance and the effects of the various interactions that are to be found within all cultures;
- it allows for the revaluation of data in relation to selected hypotheses, theories, and generalizations that are presently held about the past.

which progressivism in education appears. And it can contribute to a fuller understanding of the relationship between politics and education, between medical school and society, between local and central government, and between teacher and student.

Ex post facto research

When translated literally, *ex post facto* means 'from what is done afterwards'. Similarly, *ex post facto* research can be defined more formally as that in which the independent variable or variables have already occurred naturally and in which the researcher starts with the observation of a dependent variable or variables. He/she then studies the independent variable or variables in retrospect for their possible relationship to, and effects on, the dependent variable or variables.

Two kinds of design may be identified in *ex post facto* research—the 'correlational study' and the 'criterion group study'. The former is sometimes termed 'casual research' and the latter, 'casual-comparative research'. A correlational (or casual) study is concerned with identifying the antecedents of a present condition. As its name suggests, it involves the collection of two sets of data, one of which will be retrospective, with a view to determining the relationship between them. The basic design of such an experiment may be represented thus:

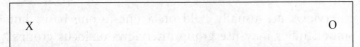

For example, let us show a relationship between the quality of a medical student undergraduate training (X) and his subsequent effectiveness as a doctor of his subject (O). Measures of the quality of a medical student college training can include grades in specific courses, overall grade average, and self-ratings, etc.

Teacher effectiveness can be assessed by indices of student performance, student knowledge, student attitudes, and judgement of experts, etc. Correlations between all measures were obtained to determine the relationship. At most, this study could show that a relationship existed, after the fact, between the quality of teacher preparation and subsequent teacher effectiveness. Where a strong relationship is found between the independent and dependent variables, three possible interpretations are open to the researcher:

- that the variable X had caused O;
- that the variable O has caused X; or
- that some third unidentified, and therefore unmeasured, variable has caused X and O.

Methods of collecting data

Having decided on how to design the research study, the next methodological decision is how to collect information. The most commonly used methods of collecting information are interviews, questionnaires, and observation.

Interviews

Interviews are usually held on a one-to-one basis, but some studies may use group interviews or focus groups. Interviews can be highly structured, semi-structured, or unstructured. The degree of structure affects the flexibility of the interview.

The use of interview in medical education research ranges from the formal interview, in which set questions are asked and the answers recorded on a standardized schedule; through less formal interviews, in which the interviewer is free to modify the sequence of questions, change the wording, explain them or add to them; to the completely informal interview where the interviewer may have a number of key issues which are raised in conversational style instead of having a set questionnaire. Beyond this point is located the non-directive interview in which the interviewer takes on a subordinate role.

Questionnaires

Questionnaires comprise a written set of questions that are answered by all respondents in a study. Several different types of questions can be used. Closed questions seek a limited response. If a range of responses can be predicted in advance—for example, eye colour—the respondent may be provided with a pre-set list of answers to choose from. At the other end of the scale, open questions allow the respondent to answer freely in their own words and are used when a more extensive response is being sought, for example an explanation. Questionnaires are often used to assess attitudes, and respondents may be asked to choose a point on a scale, either semantic or numeric, to indicate how they perceive or feel about a situation. Examples of questionnaire designs are outlined in Box 8.9.

Interview versus questionnaire

Interview is an unusual method in that it involves the gathering of data through direct verbal interaction between individuals. In this sense it differs from the questionnaire where the respondent is required to record in some way his/her responses to set questions. By way of interest, we illustrate the relative merits of the interview

---

Box 8.9   Types of questionnaire construct

Example of a closed question

Did you take the selected study module on health promotion? [ ]Yes [ ]No

Example of an open question

How would you like this course to be improved in the future? ....

Example of a rating scale

I received useful feedback. Disagree 1   2   3   4   5 Agree

---

and the questionnaire in Table 8.3. One advantage of interview is that it allows for greater depth than is the case with other methods of data collection. A disadvantage, on the other hand, is that it is prone to subjectivity and bias on the part of the interviewer.

Observation studies

Observation is a technique for collecting data through visual observation of events. It requires the nature of the data to be observable. Like the other methods of collecting data, observation schedules can be highly structured or relatively unstructured, depending on the type of information required and the nature of the observed event

The method of data collection chosen for a study should be appropriate for the type of information required. Whether the required information is quantitative or qualitative in nature is the major consideration. It would be time wasting to use unstructured interviews for essentially quantitative studies where information could be more

Table 8.3 Summary of relative merits of interview versus questionnaire

Consideration	Interview	Questionnaire
Personal need to collect data	Required	Requires a clerk
Major expense	Payment to Interviewers	Postage and printing
Opportunities for response-keying (personalization)	Extensive	Limited
Opportunities for asking	Extensive	Limited
Opportunities for probing	Possible	Difficult
Relative magnitude of data reduction	Great (because of coding)	Mainly limited to rostering
Typically the number of respondents who can be reached	Limited	Extensive
Rate of return	Good	Poor
Sources of error	Interviewer, instrument, coding, sample	Limited to instrument and sample
Overall reliability	Quite limited	Fair
Emphasis on writing skill	Limited	Extensive

Adapted from Tuckman.[9]

Table 8.4   Advantages and disadvantages of observation

Advantages	Disadvantages
Best way of recording human behaviour	Time and duration of an event may not be predictable: involves watching and waiting
Observations recorded as they occur, eliminating biased recall	Presence of observer adds a new dimension to the situation
Allows researcher to view a situation in total and in context	Presence of observer can affect people's behaviour
Observation schedules can be simple to design and use	Observations may be subject to observer bias
Observers may need little training	Observers may find themselves drawn into the situation
Open to the use of recording devices	Events may occur so rapidly it is not possible to record everything
	Little control over number of times an event will occur
	Those not wishing to be involved may object to the presence of the observer

efficiently collected through structured interviews or questionnaires. Conversely, self-completed questionnaires are generally unsuited to qualitative research: even when there is space for comments or for respondents to express ideas, the space is limited and requires respondents to have skills in articulation and literacy. The merits of the different methods of collecting data are summarized in Tables 8.3 and 8.4.

It is not always necessary to design a new data-collection tool for a research project. For example, during the literature search the researcher may discover a questionnaire that suits the intended purpose as it is acceptable to use data-collection tools that have been developed by previous researchers. It may even be preferable since the tool is more likely to have been subjected to tests for reliability and validity.

Role-playing

Role-playing has been widely used as a technique of educational research and is defined as participation in simulated social situations that are intended to throw light upon the role/rule contexts governing 'real' life social episodes.

Various role-play methods have been identified and differentiated in terms of a passive–active distinction. Thus, an individual may role-play merely by reading a description of a social episode and filling in a questionnaire about it; on the other hand, a person may role-play by being required to improvise a characterization and perform it in front of an audience. Dimensions of the role-play method are identified in Table 8.5.

A flow chart on using the role-play method in medical education research is shown in Figure 8.2.

Table 8.5   Dimensions of role-playing methods

	Form	Content
Set	Imaginary v performed	Person: self v another
Action	Scripted v improvised	Role: subject role v another role
		Context: scenario other actors
Dependent v variables	Verbal v behavioural	Audience

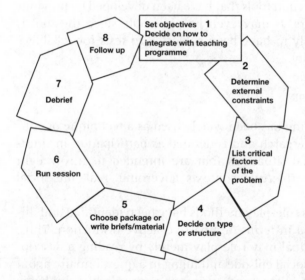

Figure 8.2   A flow chart on using the role-play method in educational research.[4]

Sampling

In any research the researcher has to identify the population under study. If a teacher wants to carry out research about students, he/she needs to decide if this means any type of student or if he is interested in a particular section of the school population. Furthermore, if he/she eventually decides what the research is actually about, for example, 'mature students', the minimum age for entering medical education or alternative criteria should be identified. If the target population is large it may not be feasible to include everyone in the research so a sample has to be selected. There are different ways of sampling and the most common ways are summarized below.[4,7]

Random sampling

This is a method that gives every member of the population a calculable chance (often equal) of being selected. It is frequently described as the method of sampling least likely to produce a bias, but sampling errors can occur by chance which can unintentionally produce bias.

Stratified sampling

This is used when the population contains subgroups and it is necessary to ensure that representatives of all groups are included, for example, students in different age bands, lecturers employed on different professional grades, hospital staff from a range of professions. Randomization within each subgroup can be applied.

Systematic sampling

This involves taking the nth name on a list, such as every third person or every tenth. Unless the list is arranged randomly, the sample will not be random. This approach may eliminate certain members of the population who may have a perspective, which is useful to the study, but go unnoticed, for example, taking the first-named member of the household from an electoral roll will almost certainly eliminate the younger members of the population.

Cluster sampling

This is used when the population is diversely spread over a geographical area, where for various reasons it is preferable to include groups of subjects from several sites rather than randomly selecting the whole sample from the whole population. An example of this would be: to investigate the grades of final year medical students nationally, the sample could select a sample of medical students in one city in each of the local regions of the UK.

Convenience or incidental sampling

This method utilizes readily available subjects and is often used in qualitative projects and hypothesis generating. The sample may not be representative of the population as a whole and the results may not be able to be generalized; for example, students selected from one learning resource.

Sequential sampling

The size of the sample is not pre-set. The researcher collects data from each subject in turn until he/she is satisfied that there is no new information for collection of the topic is saturated. It is used mostly in qualitative research, for example, in setting up a new curriculum, potential students are asked what they would want until no new ideas emerge.

Purposive sampling

Subjects are selected because they have certain characteristics, for example, all the final year students in the medical school.

Ethical issues

In trying to access the sample, the researcher has to consider how this can practically be achieved and whose permission must be sought. For example, access to students normally requires permission from the responsible school officer or the university. Access to lecturers requires permission from their Head of Department. By seeking permission to contact the sample group, the researcher is also more likely to secure practical help and advice to access subjects.

The researcher must also consider any ethical implications of the research. At the very least this involves issues of confidentiality and anonymity, but there may be other factors to consider which, unless resolved, could potentially have negative implications for the subjects directly or indirectly. For example, research which tests the effectiveness of new teaching approaches may eventually show that the new approach is better than the old, but in order to find out, it may be necessary to withhold the established teaching method from a sample of group of students. Any risks or issues associated with this should be carefully assessed. The researcher should seek advice and, if necessary, formal permission to undertake the study from the relevant authority.

The pilot study

Once the researcher is ready to undertake the study he/she should carry out a small pilot study to check that the methodology has been thought through correctly. The pilot is the miniature study and gives the researcher an opportunity to identify any problems and to modify the research method before embarking on the main study.

The pilot study enables the researcher to check the following:

- the accessibility of the sample group;
- the likely response rate;
- whether or not the data-collection tool provides the depth, range, and quality of information required.

If problems are detected at the pilot study stage the researcher has the opportunity to make revisions before undertaking the main study. This increases the likelihood that the data collected in the main study will be usable.

Data collection

Once the methodology has been thought through and the method of data collection has been piloted, the researcher reaches the stage of conducting the interviews, sending out the questionnaires, or recording observations. For many researchers, this is the most exciting or enjoyable part of the research process. After what can sometimes be weeks or months of planning for developing the research idea, reviewing the literature, designing the research method, the researcher starts to investigate the topic through the collection of original data.

Data analysis

This is the next stage of the research process, when the researcher reviews the data collected and systematically analyses the responses of subjects. Up to this point every participant's responses form a separate record. Combining all these separate records into one and providing an overview produces the results of a research study.

Data are described, summarized and, if quantitative in nature, statistically analysed in order to produce the results of the study. The techniques employed in data analysis are dependent on the type of information collected, the research design and the design of the data-collection tool. As we have already seen, qualitative and quantitative data are very different in content and require very different approaches. Qualitative data is analysed by reading respondents' comments (questionnaires and interview transcripts), or by listening to their comments (tape-recorded interviews) or by reviewing their behaviour (observation) or by watching their actions (role-play). The range of responses is described and examples of behaviour or narrative are used to illustrate both the typicality and diversity of responses.

Quantitative data are analysed by counting the frequency with which certain features occur among participants' responses. The summarized data can then be subjected to a variety of statistical measures to identify patterns or trends (descriptive statistics) and to assess what inferences can be made from the data about the general population (inferential statistics).

If the research project is a small-scale study with data collection from a small sample and the researcher does not want to carry out sophisticated statistical analysis, it should be possible to analyse the data by hand. If not, then it is advisable to use computerized software packages (for example, SPSS, Minitab, Microsoft Excel). They require the data to be inserted manually, although the computer does the hard work of calculating and comparing the results.

Drawing conclusions

When the data have been analysed and a full set of results has been produced, the researcher reviews the results and considers them in the context of previous knowledge. This final stage of the research process contains three key elements:

- discussing the findings;
- identifying the limitations of the study;
- making recommendations for further research and for practice.

The results are considered in light of the original research problem. If this was stated as an aim, the researcher discusses the extent to which the aim was achieved. If the research problem was stated as a question, the researcher considers whether the research study has provided an answer. If a hypothesis was used, the researcher has to decide whether it can be accepted or rejected according to the results.

In considering the overall strengths and weaknesses of the study design, the results identify the limitations of the research project. For example, the size or selection of the sample may limit the generalizability of the results, or the depth and breadth of data may limit the conclusions that can be drawn. It is important that the limitations of a study are always recognized, as readers should take them into consideration when deciding whether or not to act on the results of the study.

Finally, consideration is given to how the results could be applied to practice. At the beginning of this chapter it was stated that research is intended to add to the body of knowledge, but if the limitations are extensive, the research will have limited value. Caution should therefore be exercised in recommending changes to current teaching practice or making unrealistic claims about the extent to which knowledge can be informed by the findings. In this case it is more appropriate for the researcher to identify the need for further research and to make recommendations about the direction that the research could take.

Conclusion

This chapter has provided a brief overview of the research process in medical education. We have looked at the sequence of steps taken by researchers as they plan a research project, undertake the project, and make sense of the findings. The information on methodology has shown that there are different types of research and that the choice of method depends on the research problem, the type of information needed and practical matters such as the time and resources available to carry out the research. Depending on previous knowledge, the chapter may have acted as an introduction or as a reminder of the main elements of the research process.

References

1. Harden RM. Approaches to research in medical education. *Medical Education* 1986; **20**: 522–31.
2. Mouly GJ. *Educational Research: the Art and Science of Investigation.* Boston: Allyn & Bacon, 1978.
3. Hancock BC. An introduction to research methodology. In:Wilson A, Williams M, Hancock B, eds. *Research Approaches in Primary Care.* Oxford: Radcliffe Medical Press, 2000.
4. Osonnaya C, Osonnaya K. *Research Methods in Medical Education.* London: Kingscos Medical Publishers, 2000.
5. Carter Y, Thomas C, eds. *Research Methods in Primary Care.* Oxford: Radcliffe Medical Press, 1997.
6. Irby DM. Shifting paradigms of research in medical education. *Academic Medicine* 1990; **65**(10): 622–3.
7. Cohen L, Mannion D. *Research Method in Education.* London: Routledge, 1994.

8.   Halpin D, Croll P, Redman K. Teachers' perceptions of the effects of in service education. *British Educational Research Journal* 1990; **16**(2): 163–77.
9.   Tuckman BW. *Conducting Educational Research.* New York: Harcourt Brace Jovanovich, 1972.

Further reading

The following books are recommended for their review of the trends and issues in research in medical education and their application in teaching and learning in primary care.

Calder J. *Survey Research Methods.* ASME Medical Education Research Booklet No. 6. Edinburgh: Association for the Study of Medical Education, 1998. ISBN 0 904473 23 6.

Carter Y, Thomas C, eds. *Research Methods in Primary Care.* Oxford: Radcliffe Medical Press, 1997. ISBN 1 85775 198 1.

Cohen L, Mannion L. *Research Methods in Education,* 4th edn. London: Routledge, 1994. ISBN 0 415 10235 9.

Fleming WG. *The Observation of Educational Events.* ASME Medical Education Research Booklet No. 5. Edinburgh: Association for the Study of Medical Education, 1998. ISBN 0 904473 13 9.

Gantley M, Harding G, Kumar S, Tissier J. An introduction to qualitative methods for health professionals. In: *Master Classes in Primary Care Research No.1.* Eds: Carter Y, Shaw S, Thomas C. London: Royal College of General Practitioners, 1999. ISBN 0 85084 246 8.

McColl E, Thomas R. The use and design of questionnaires. In: *Master Classes in Primary Care Research No.2.* Eds: Carter Y, Shaw S, Thomas C. London: Royal College of General Practitioners, 2000. ISBN 0 85084 247 6.

Osonnaya C, Osonnaya K. Research Methods in Medical Education. London: Kingscos Medical Publishers, 2000. ISBN 1 903823 01 3.

Underwood M, Hannaford P, Slowther A. Randomised Controlled Trials and Multi-Centre Research. In: *Master Classes in Primary Care Research No.4.* Eds: Carter Y, Shaw S, Thomas C. London: Royal College of General Practitioners, 2000. ISBN 0 85084 251 4.

Woodward CA. Questionnaire Construction and Questionnaire Writing for Research in Medical Education. ASME Medical Education Research Booklet No. 4. Edinburgh: Association for the Study of Medical Education, 1998. ISBN 0 904473 10 4.

9 Clinical effectiveness and evidence-based primary care

YVONNE CARTER AND
MAGGIE FALSHAW

Clinical effectiveness

In recent years research and development (R&D) have had a high profile in the provision of health care. As a result, clinical effectiveness has become a key topic for primary care practitioners. This chapter examines the development of evidence-based practice and its relationship to primary care and considers the links between health services, research and development, and education and training (Figure 9.1).

In its December 1997 White Paper, *The New NHS:*

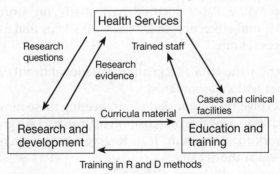

Figure 9.1 Links between the three systems.

Box 9.1   Clinical effectiveness framework

- Clear link to NHS R&D strategy
- Ensure the latest evidence about effectiveness is readily available
- Use of clinical guidelines
- Use of clinical audit
- Development of health outcome indicators
- Change clinical practice
- Monitor effects of change

Modern and Dependable,[1] the government stated that it would put quality at the heart of the NHS. It set out an ambitious and far-reaching 10-year programme of modernization, describing how the internal market would be replaced by a system of integrated care, based on partnership and driven by performance. The document promised early, visible improvements to the quality of service people experience in their own homes, at their GP surgery or health centre, and in hospital.

The White Paper focused particularly on structures, quality, and efficiency and six key principles underlie the changes set out:

- renew the NHS as a genuinely national health service (set national standards);
- devolve the responsibility for meeting these new standards to a local level (creation of primary care groups);
- work in partnership (e.g. forging stronger links with local authorities);
- improve efficiency so that all money is spent to maximize patient care;

- shift the focus to quality of care ensuring excellence is guaranteed to *all* patients;
- make the NHS more open and accountable to the public.

Under the new arrangements, health authorities now take the lead in drawing up 3-year health improvement programmes and have responsibility for improving overall health and reducing health inequalities. Following publication of *Our Healthier Nation*,[2] health authorities have a duty to improve the health of their population.

In *A First Class Service: Quality in the New NHS*,[3] published in 1998, the Government set out in some detail how it intended to implement the changes in England and asked for views about how the objectives could best be met. The document emphasizes the importance of the active participation of clinical professionals and patients throughout the NHS. The main elements of the proposals are:

- clear national standards for services and treatments, through evidence-based national service frameworks and a new National Institute for Clinical Excellence;
- local delivery of high-quality health care, through clinical governance underpinned by modernized professional self-regulation and extended lifelong learning (see Chapter 4);
- effective monitoring of progress through a new Commission of Health Improvement, a Framework for Assessing Performance in the NHS and a new national survey of patient and user experience.

The establishment of primary care groups in 1999 has set a new agenda for service development and research in the NHS. *The New NHS*,[1] clinical effectiveness indicators and action on clinical audit place at the centre of the primary care agenda the delivery of health care that is research based, of proven efficacy, and audited. All areas

---

Box 9.2   The new NHS

- National services—national frameworks
- Local responsibility—patients' needs
- Partnership—new duties
- Efficiency—incentives
- Excellence—local and national
- Public confidence—openness

Box 9.3   Clinical governance

- Quality improvement, e.g. clinical audit
- Good practice systematically disseminated
- Adverse events detected, openly investigated, and lessons learned
- Poor clinical performance dealt with
- Professional development programmes aligned

---

of the health service are being encouraged to develop a culture based on enquiry and the use of research evidence to inform practice. Evidence-based health care enables primary care workers to base decisions about diagnosis, treatment, and management of patients on the best evidence available.

Using the best possible information to help in making clinical decisions is at the heart of evidence-based practice. Evidence-based health care and clinical governance aim to promote health care that is effective—and that does more good than harm. This can only be achieved if relevant research findings and valid guideline recommendations are incorporated into practice. The research literature, however, varies in its degree of accuracy and completeness.

For GPs to make properly informed decisions about care, it is essential that they have access to the best possible, most complete and up-to-date information they can find. Most people do not have the time to track down all the relevant research studies when trying to answer a clinical problem. Once the studies have been identified, it can also be both difficult and confusing to assess the quality and the sometimes conflicting results from different research studies.

Research findings can influence decisions at many levels—in planning care for individual patients, in the development of practice guidelines, in improving the delivery of education and training (see Chapter 8) and in commissioning health care when developing strategies for health promotion and preventive health. It can also be used in the development of policy—at a local practice, PCG/T, community trust, or at a national level. But research findings can only play this role if research knowledge is translated into action.

Development of evidence-based health care

The concept of evidence-based health care is not new but its development has been highlighted over the last 10 years. Much of the impetus comes from within medicine itself. Evidence-based medicine, or EBM as it has been commonly called, has also been an international phenomenon. Sackett and colleagues in McMaster University in Canada developed EBM as a method of promoting lifelong learning.[4] More recently, evidence-based health care has developed in a number of centres in the UK including the development of the NHS Centre for Reviews and Dissemination at the University of York and the UK Cochrane Centre in Oxford.

Evidence-based health care has been described as 'the conscientious, explicit and judicious use of current best evidence in making decisions about the care of individual patients'[5]. The practice of evidence-based medicine means integrating individual clinical expertise with the best available external clinical evidence from systematic research. Consider evidence-based medicine as primarily an educational strategy: it is about *using* research, rather than *doing* research.

In order to practise evidence-based care, we not only need to have the evidence, we also need to know how good the evidence is and whether it is appropriate for our patient populations. Traditionally most medical research, particularly using a randomized controlled trial design, has been based in hospital settings. There are differences between patients in hospital and the general population. If we take the example of patients with diabetes, those in the general population are likely to have fewer complications and their diabetes is likely to be better controlled than is the case with patients with diabetes who are admitted to hospital. The diagnosis may be the same but there will be important differences in their health status. Because of these differences, research conducted solely with hospital patients will indicate different treatment regimens and thresholds than research whose subjects include patients at home.

The importance of primary care as a setting for clinical research has been recognized.[6,7] Taken together, these two reports, published in 1997, the National Working Group on R&D in primary care, and the Medical Research Council's topic review in primary health care, have set the scene for a series of steps towards achieving the potential of an integrated clinical academic career structure in primary care. The Mant report[6] has been of relevance to all professional groups working in primary care and set specific objectives including increasing the recruitment, development, and retention of R&D leaders in primary care. In putting the case for supporting R&D in primary care, Mant explains that over 90% of contact between the population and the NHS take place in primary care. Most minor illness is treated entirely in primary care and most serious disease presents first in primary care. In addition, chronic illness is increasingly managed in primary care.

Primary care clinicians have responsibility in making decisions about diagnosis, referral to secondary care, and prescribing medication. An evidence-based approach is important for all three. The need for a firm knowledge base is as important in primary as in secondary care (see Chapter 13). Much of the evidence required by primary care can only be obtained through research that is conducted in primary care settings which involve primary care practitioners and their patients.

Opportunities to engage in primary care research and development are growing and the scope for those wishing to become involved is finally widening. The Culyer report[8] took steps to redress the underdevelopment of primary care research in relation to that in other sectors, by increasing the proportion of NHS R&D funding available for primary care. Infrastructure funding for research active practices and the evolution of primary care research networks should both help to improve the research capacity and blur some of the boundaries between academic departments and clinical practice.

In 1999, the Central Research and Development Committee, which advises the Director of Research and Development at the Department of Health on the strategic framework and priorities for the use of the NHS R&D Levy, established a Strategic Review Sub-group, to review this framework. Five topic working groups were established in the following areas to facilitate this review: ageing, cancer, cardiovascular disease and stroke, mental health, and primary care. The report on primary care[9] recommended that research should address the following areas:

- the demand for quality;
- the importance of partnership;
- the problem of inequality;
- the generalist role; and
- technological advances.

We are beginning to see an increase in primary-care-based research, which is in turn leading to an increase in an evidence base for primary care decision making. Translating research evidence into research practice will facilitate the promotion of effective health care. Lomas[10] described three stages in the flow of research into practice: diffusion, dissemination, and implementation.

Practising evidence-based heath care—putting evidence into practice

David Sackett has defined evidence-based medicine as:

a process of life-long, self-directed learning in which caring for one's own patients creates the need for clinically important information about diagnosis, prognosis and therapy, and other clinical and health care issues.[5]

There is a need to:

- convert these needs into answerable questions;
- track down efficiently the best evidence to answer them;
- critically appraise that evidence for its validity and usefulness;

- apply the results of this appraisal in their clinical practice;
- evaluate our own performance.

Formulating the question

It is important to define questions in a way that is relevant to the problem at hand, and to phrase them to facilitate searching for a precise answer. One way of focusing questions is to think of them as having four parts:

- a patient or problem
- an intervention or exposure
- a comparison, if relevant
- a clinical outcome.

Questions typically arise in one of the following areas of clinical work:

- *clinical evidence*: how to gather clinical findings properly and interpret them soundly;
- *diagnosis*: how to select and interpret diagnostic tests;
- *therapy*: how to select treatments that do more good than harm;
- *prognosis*: how to anticipate the patient's likely course;
- *prevention*: how to screen for and reduce the risk of disease;
- *education*: how to teach yourself and a patient what is needed.

Tracking down the evidence

When carrying out research, access to and competence in using electronic databases such as Medline is important. It is important to remember to go for efficiency (reading a well conducted review or guideline is better than sifting through many individual studies). Databases of secondary sources are increasingly becoming available. The National Electronic Library for Health (NeLH) provides a gateway to the Cochrane Library, Clinical Evidence and other evidence-based information.

Clinical guidelines have been promoted as a means to ensure that research evidence is put into practice and this has been supported by the NHS Executive.[11] Criteria have been published for the successful development and implementation of clinical guidelines[12] and information on effective treatment has been made available to NHS staff through the publication of the *Effective Health Care* bulletins and a number of other sources outlined in Box 9.9. The National Institute for Clinical Excellence (NICE) guidelines are readily available.

Research evidence is often quoted in the general media. It is often a criterion of funding that lay summaries of research findings are made available to the public. Patients often raise concerns about reports in the press, particularly if they have experienced the condition or procedures reported. NeLH includes the Hitting the Headlines Service. This contains rapid critical appraisal, conducted by Centre for Reviews and Dissemination at the University of York,

---

Box 9.4   Improving clinical effectiveness with clinical guidelines

- Nationally endorsed
- Research based
- Cost of interventions included
- Multidisciplinary
- Patient perspective
- Ethical consideration

of research reported in the national press. The short reviews include a summary of the article and an evaluation of the evidence. The latter looks at where the evidence comes from, the objectives of the study, the study methodology, its conclusions and their reliability. The review includes references and links to consumer information.

Applying the results

Many of the more sterile arguments about how evidence is applied to individual patients lose their force if the primary goal of the exercise is to make a clinical decision not savage a paper!

Evaluating performance

Using an evidence-based approach to setting standards is a possible way to make audit more interesting, and including this step is likely to enhance the educational benefits of EBM.

How do primary care clinicians integrate the best available external clinical evidence with their individual clinical expertise?

The case study illustrates the steps outlined above.

Case Study

Sharon Browne, a 35-year-old woman, attends evening surgery. She was diagnosed with Ménière's disease 4 years ago. She has a history of attacks every 2–3 months when she experiences vertigo, hearing loss, and tinnitus lasting a few hours. When the diagnosis was first made, the consultant prescribed frusemide, which she now gets on repeat prescription from you. Sharon says she doesn't want another prescription as the water tablets make her feel awful and she wants to stop taking them. Sharon is a non-smoker, has adjusted her diet to reduce her salt and fat intake, and takes regular exercise. She's been your patient for 6 years and you have got to know her well during that time. Although you know that diuretics are part of the usual treatment for Ménière's, you agree to read up on this and ask her to make an appointment for the following week when her current prescription runs out. She agrees to continue the frusemide until then.

Framing the question

Is frusemide an effective treatment for the management of Ménière's disease?

Searching for the best available evidence

Evidence about the most effective way of achieving these changes can be obtained from a number of sources as shown in Box 9.8.

Box 9.8   Sources of evidence

- Patient narrative
- Own experience
- Colleagues
- Experts
- Decision support—PRODIGY, Mentor, etc.
- Evidence-based databases and reviews
- Research papers

Patient narrative
Patients' experiences, fears, and health beliefs are important when planning risk reduction or other interventions. Apart from Ménière's, Sharon has good health. She is a non-smoker, she exercises regularly, and she has a healthy diet. She takes her medication routinely.

Your own experience
Experience about strategies and approaches that have or have not worked in the past are an important source of evidence. Any prior knowledge of the individual patient will also play a part. You know that diuretics are included routinely in the management of Ménière's. You feel that you have a good relationship with Sharon.

Colleagues and experts
Colleagues and experts are further sources of evidence. As a partner or non-principal, your GP and practice nurse colleagues will also have useful advice and opinions for you to consider. The hospital consultant sees more patients with Ménière's than you do and she says that she always starts them on diuretics.

Decision support software
Decision support software, such as PRODIGY and Mentor, may provide sources of clinical evidence for this issue. You have Mentor 2 on your practice computer and check it for sources of evidence about Ménière's disease. You find a link to a Bandolier article, to a research paper, and to patient information leaflets.

Secondary sources of evidence
Bandolier searched the literature for treatment of Ménière's disease. A review of Medline 1978–1995 is reported.[13] This reported one trial which included diuretics.

It found that they were effective in controlling vertigo but had no effect on hearing. The article concludes that apart from betahistine, 'there seems little good evidence for effective treatments of Ménière's disease'.

Mentor also listed three research papers, one of which looks promising.[14] You search the electronic BMJ http://www.bmj.com to get a full text version of the paper. Saeed conducted a literature review of the diagnosis and treatment of Ménière's disease. Saeed reports that the use of diuretics had a historical rather than scientific basis, as the findings from the few controlled studies that had been conducted were conflicting and the placebo effect was clinically significant. He concludes that betahistine, with or without a diuretic, constitutes the favoured means of providing maintenance medical treatment.

Putting evidence into practice

When Sharon attends for her next appointment you explain that you have searched the research literature and although diuretics are usually included in the treatment for Ménière's disease there is no hard evidence of their effectiveness. As the diuretics are making her feel nauseous you suggest that she stops taking them, and agrees to keep a diary of attacks and the symptoms she experiences during them and to telephone you if she feels any other symptoms.

A growing number of evidence-based databases can be drawn upon to assist the practice of clinically effective and evidence-based health care (Box 9.9).

Finding and appraising the evidence yourself

If you are unable to find a rapid appraisal or evidence summary for your question, or if you are undertaking a research or educational project, you will need to find and appraise the papers yourself.

Box 9.9 Evidence-based websites

Academic sites

- University of Oxford: Health Services Research Unit: http//hsru.dphpc.ox.ac.uk/research.html. Includes overviews of systematic reviews of effectiveness.
- University of London: Institute of Education: Social Science Research Unit EPI Centre: http://www.ioe.ac.uk/ssru/ra epi.html. The EPI-Centre aims to promote evidence-based practice and practice-based research in health promotion and social interventions, to promote lay involvement in all stages of health research from setting the agenda to sharing and making use of the findings. The website provides a résumé of the work of the EPI Centre and a list of contacts. The list of current projects gives a listing of the current projects on the evaluation of interventions with contact details.

Electronic journals

- Bandolier: http://www.jr2.ox.ac.uk/Bandolier. Bandolier is produced monthly in Oxford for the NHS R&D Directorate. It contains bullet points (hence Bandolier) of evidence-based medicine.
- Cochrane Library: http://www.update-software.com/ccweb/. UK Cochrane Centre Library.
- http://www.york.ac.uk/inst/crd/cochlib.html. Training materials in Word and PowerPoint on efficient use of the Cochrane Library.
- Effective Health Care Bulletins. http://www.york.ac.uk/inst/crd/ehcb.html. Effective Health Care (EHC) is a bi-monthly bulletin for decision makers, which examines the effectiveness of a variety of health care interventions. EHC bulletins are produced by CRD

continued

and published by The Royal Society of Medicine Press Ltd.

- Effectiveness Matters: http://www.york.ac.uk/inst/crd/em.html. Effectiveness Matters is produced to complement EHC, and provides updates on the effectiveness of important health interventions for practitioners and decision makers in the NHS. It covers topics in a shorter and more journalistic style, summarizing the results of high-quality systematic reviews.

Learning resources

- CASP (Critical Appraisal Skills Programme): http://www.his.ox.ac.uk/casp/. CASP is a UK project that aims to help health service decision makers develop skills in the critical appraisal of evidence about effectiveness, in order to promote the delivery of evidence-based health care. This website gives background information about CASP and provides contact details.

Other NHS and UK official sites

- National Institute for Clinical Effectiveness—NICE (UK): http://www.nice.org.uk. NICE is a new Special Health Authority with a remit to systematically appraise health interventions before they are introduced in the health service. It will offer clinicians and health professionals clear guidelines on which treatments work best for patients, and which do not. This website contains information about NICE, related news, links, FAQs and other information.
- National Electronic Library for Health (NeLH): http://www.nhs.uk/nelh/. This site provides evaluated health information for practitioners and the public. Hitting the Headlines provides brief appraisals of health research recently quoted in the popular media. The site also includes links to Medline and

continued

Cochrane, and to an electronic version of Clinical Evidence.
- NHS Centre for Reviews and Dissemination, University of York: http://www.york.ac.uk/inst/crd/welcome.html. The NHS Centre for Reviews and Dissemination exists to provide the NHS with information on the effectiveness of treatments and the delivery and organization of health care. Their Database of Abstracts of Reviews of Effectiveness (DARE) covers the published literature on effectiveness of health-care interventions, while the NHS Economic Evaluation database concentrates on the economic aspects.
- UK Cochrane Centre. Supports the NHS Research and Development Programme and is part of the worldwide Cochrane Collaboration.

The increase in primary care research is reflected in the number of papers published in peer review journals. Electronic databases are a useful tool for finding appropriate research papers. Medline is an international database of biomedical and associated health literature compiled by the National Library of Medicine in the United States. It is often the first database clinicians search when looking for papers.

Medline can be accessed through the BMA website: http://www.bma.co.uk/, through NeLH, through Medical School libraries and some PCG/T websites. It can also be accessed through http://biomednet.com.

A clinical librarian can help in the development of a search strategy.

Limitations of Medline

Finding quality evidence to support patient care is difficult.[15,16] Although a Medline search is a useful place to start to look for references addressing clinical issues, it is not exhaustive. Medline has over 9.5 million references from 3900 journals but it is geared towards American publications. A number of important journals such as *Health Service Journal, Health Education Journal, Quality in Health Care* and *New Scientist* are not listed on Medline.

Even when the references are on Medline, you aren't certain to pick them up. Sometimes the problems are caused by inadequacies in indexing. In general, only 50% of the trials in Medline can be found by even the best electronic searchers. A study found that 18% of randomized controlled trials (RCTs) were found by experienced clinical searching; 52% with someone with optimal Medline searching skills; and 94% were found through hand searching.

The Cochrane Collaboration is working to overcome this information gap by hand searching journals and incorporating any trials that are found into Medline. Cochrane Reviews are now listed on Medline.

Although a Medline search will not be complete, it is still likely to give references which aren't relevant for your specific question. You will need to discard these. Some references can be discarded by looking at the title of the paper. However, you may still be left with articles that aren't relevant. Skim reading the abstract of the articles will give an idea which ones are worth keeping in your list and which you should discard. This is not foolproof, but can help you discard some articles that aren't appropriate for your question.

The more experience you have of Medline searching, the more skilful you become at it, and your searches will be more complete and precise. Once you have found papers that may address the question, you need to read the papers and appraise their quality. You need to judge the research evidence.

Appraising the evidence

For those who wish to appraise the evidence themselves, we recommend a simplified approach based on *The User's Guides to the Medical Literature*.[17-25] In these guides, three questions are asked of any study:

- Is the study valid?
- What are the results?
- Can I use the results in caring for my patients?

The ways in which validity is determined and the results interpreted will obviously depend on whether the study considers diagnosis, therapy, prognosis, etc., but these three simple questions provide a framework for tackling any study.

Critical appraisal

The three main methodologies used in primary care research are quantitative research, including RCTs and cohort studies; qualitative research, and evaluation of cost effectiveness. Appraisal tools for each of these have been developed:

- http://www.public-health.org.uk/Casp/rct.html;
- http://www.public-health.org.uk/Casp/quantitative. html;
- http://www.public-health.org.uk/Casp/economic. html.

Conclusion

Delivering health care that is clinically effective and based on research evidence is important. The increase in support for primary-care-based research encourages the development of a research culture within primary care. If we return to Figure 9.1 we can see that research questions arise from the delivery of health services. The role of research and development (R&D) is to help find the research evidence to answer those questions. To practise clinical effectiveness this evidence has to be incorporated into clinical practice. Education and training are needed to enable clinicians to develop skills to enable them to conduct primary care research and to judge the research of others. The appraisal of the evidence is fed back into the delivery of health care. Research evidence has a role in the development of materials for use in undergraduate and postgraduate education. Recipients of the education and training courses are involved in the delivery of health care services.

References

1. Secretary of State for Health. *The New NHS: Modern and Dependable.* London: Department of Health, 1997.
2. Secretary of State for Health. *Our Healthier Nation.* London: The Stationery Office, 1999.
3. Secretary of State for Health. *A First Class Service: Quality in the New NHS* London: Department of Health, 1998.
4. Sackett D, Rosenburg W, Gray J, Haynes B, Richardson WS. Evidence based medicine: what and what it isn't. *British Medical Journal* 1996; **289**: 587–90.
5. Sackett DL. *Evidence-based Medicine; How to Teach and Practise EBM.* Edinburgh: Churchill Livingstone, 1997.
6. Mant D. *R&D in Primary Care: National Working Group Report.* Leeds: Department of Health, 1997.
7. Medical Research Council. *MRC Topic Review: Primary Health Care 1997.* London: Medical Research Council, 1997.
8. National Health Service Research and Development Task Force. *Supporting Research and Development in the NHS.* London: HMSO, 1994.
9. Clarke M. *NHS R+D Strategic Review Primary Care.* Leeds: Department of Health, 1999.
10. Lomas J. Diffusion, dissemination and implementation—who should do what. *Annals of the New York Academy of Sciences* 1993; **703**: 226–35.

11. NHS Executive. *Promoting Clinical Effectiveness. A Framework for Action In and Through the NHS*. Leeds: NHS Executive, 1996.

12. Nuffield Institute for Health. *Implementing Clinical Guidelines. Effective Health Care*, Bulletin 8. Leeds: University of Leeds, 1994.

13. Tinnitus and Ménière's update. **Bandolier** 2000; 74–2.

14. Saeed SR. Diagnosis and treatment of Ménière's disease. *British Medical Journal* 1998; **316**: 368–72.

15. McKibbon KA, Walker-Dilks CJ. The quality and impact of MEDLINE searches performed by end users. *Health Libraries Review* 1995; **12**: 191–200.

16. Haynes RB, McKibbon KA, Walker CJ, *et al*. Online access to MEDLINE in clinical settings. A study of use and usefulness. *Annals of Internal Medicine* 1990; **112**: 78–84.

17. Oxman AD, Sackett DL, Guyatt GH. Users' guides to the medical literature. I. How to get started. The Evidence-Based Medicine Working Group. *Journal of the American Medical Association* 1993; **270**: 2093–5.

18. Guyatt GH, Sackett DL, Cook DJ. Users' guides to the medical literature. II. How to use an article about therapy or prevention. A. Are the results of the study valid? Evidence-Based Medicine Working Group. *Journal of the American Medical Association* 1993; **270**: 2598–601.

19. Jaeschke R, Guyatt G, Sackett DL. Users' guides to the medical literature. III. How to use an article about a diagnostic test. A. Are the results of the study valid? Evidence-Based Medicine Working Group. *Journal of the American Medical Association* 1994; **271**: 389–91.

20. Jaeschke R, Guyatt GH, Sackett DL. Users' guides to the medical literature. III. How to use an article about a diagnostic test. B. What are the results and will they help me in caring for my patients? The Evidence-Based Medicine Working Group. *Journal of the American Medical Association* 1994; **271**: 703–7.

21. Levine M, Walter S, Lee H, Haines T, Holbrook A, Moyer V. Users' guides to the medical literature. IV. How to use an article about harm. Evidence-Based Medicine Working Group. *Journal of the American Medical Association* 1994; **271**: 1615–19.

22. Laupacis A, Wells G, Richardson WS, Tugwell P. Users' guides to the medical literature. V. How to use an article about prognosis. Evidence-Based Medicine Working Group. *Journal of the American Medical Association* 1994; **272**: 234–7.

23. Oxman AD, Cook DJ, Guyatt GH. Uses' guides to the medical literature. VI. How to use an overview. Evidence-Based Medicine Working Group. *Journal of the American Medical Association* 1994; **272**: 1367–71.

24. Richardson WS, Detsky AS. Users' guides to the medical literature. VII. How to use a clinical decision analysis. A. Are the results of the study valid? Evidence-Based Medicine Working Group. *Journal of the American Medical Association* 1995; **273**: 1292–5.

25. Hayward RS, Wilson MC, Tunis SR, Bass EB, Guyatt G. Users' guides to the medical literature. VIII. How to use clinical practice guidelines. A. Are the recommendations valid? The Evidence-Based Medicine Working Group. *Journal of the American Medical Association* 1995; **274**: 570–4.

Further reading

BMJ Publishing Group. Clinical Evidence. A Compendium of the Best Available Evidence for Effective Health Care. London: BMJ Publishing Group, 1999.

Carter YH, Falshaw M, eds. *Evidence-based Primary Health Care. An Open Learning Programme.* Oxford: Radcliffe Medical Press, 1998.

Chambers R. *Clinical Effectiveness Made Easy: First Thoughts on Clinical Governance.* Oxford: Radcliffe Medical Press. 1998.

Eldridge S, Ashby D. Statistical concepts. In: Carter Y, Shaw S, Thomas C, eds. *Master Classes in Primary Case Research No.3.* London: Royal College of General Practitioners, 2000. ISBN 0 85084 250 6

Thomas C. Critical appraisal of the literature. In: Carter YH, Thomas C, eds. *Research Methods in Primary Care.* Oxford: Radcliffe Medical Press, 1996.

10 Information, learning and new technologies

ALEX JAMIESON AND
TONY RENNISON

Background

Alex Jamieson is a GP with 12 years' experience in Continuing Education for GPs both as a GP Tutor and as an Associate Dean of Postgraduate GP Education. Tony Rennison is an Information Technology specialist who has considerable experience as a teacher in the use of primary care computer systems by health-care professionals. He is also the author of a book on the subject,[1] and is a non-GP who is an Associate Dean of Postgraduate GP Education.

A 'rapid appraisal' of the current use of information technology by GPs in addressing their continuing education was commissioned for this chapter and was conducted by Ruth Pinder,[2] an experienced qualitative researcher. Extracts from Dr Pinder's work are reproduced with the permission of the author.

This chapter discusses the use of information and communications technology (ICT) in GP Continuing Professional Development (CPD) both in the non-clinical and in the clinical environment. The use of new technologies in the non-clinical environment is discussed in relation to learning processes and the design of educational resources. The use of information management and technology (IM&T) in the clinical environment is addressed from an educational standpoint.

Introduction

Most articles and other texts published on the subject of new technologies begin with a statement like the one below:

Technology continues to progress at a rate such that most individuals have difficulty maintaining a current level of understanding or comprehension for its capabilities.[3]

We are all in a sense overwhelmed by information both on and in the technological revolution taking place around us. Anyone who acts on their own curiosity in the field of information technology and education is overwhelmed in turn by the large number of publications which address the current issues and debates. A search on a publications database for current publications in the field of education and ICT, IM&T, and similar terms, produces a list of literally hundreds of books, many published in the last 3 years, and many more in the process of publication. Similarly, a search for journal articles in educational databases produces a list of hundreds of articles addressing new technology issues.

The theoretical debate in the field of new technology and education centres largely on the following:

- first, how to produce educational materials and manage educational processes using new technologies;
- second, whether or not such educational materials and processes enhance learning in comparison with traditional methodologies; and
- third, how best to utilize the potential for learners of new kinds of learning networks.

In practice, the most immediate way in which new technology impinges on learning for GPs is in the clinical setting, in the fundamental use of primary care clinical systems, and it is from here that the most immediately useful changes to practice are realized.

This chapter discusses, first, the theoretical issues which surround learning processes and educational media using new technologies primarily in the non-clinical context, then discusses in detail the various modes of facilitated learning which can take place in the clinical context. Clearly there is some overlap between clinical and non-clinical contexts in the use of new technologies, but we have maintained the separation to clarify the issues.

The use of new technologies in continuing professional development (CPD)

The CPD requirements which GPs now face in terms of the completion of a Personal Development Plan (PDP) as part of a Practice Professional Development Plan (PPDP), and the forthcoming requirement for all doctors to assemble a portfolio of evidence of learning progress to prepare for revalidation, encourage reflection on experience and dialogue with colleagues, and allow us to exercise considerable learner autonomy. We can thus make our own choices and set our own agendas in the context of our learning.

When we start to use new technologies, however, such as are exemplified by CD-ROM/DVD or web-based applications, we are much more dependent in the majority of cases on the teacher/designer, the person who has been involved in the initial design of the learning process we are undertaking. This mimics earlier more dependent learning experiences such as are remembered from school or higher education. This clearly contrasts with the adult learning experience we have in CPD where we are often discussing learning experiences on an equal footing with colleagues, but for new technologies, as we have explained, it has relevance, especially for the non-clinical environment.

This and the following section discuss the use of new technologies in facilitated learning processes (processes where there is a designated teacher/designer) and then analyse the characteristics of the different available media in relation to an ideal facilitated learning process.

In the debate surrounding the use of new technologies in learning, the question arises: 'Does the new technology bestow an added benefit to the learner?' (Chambers,[4] page 5), in contrast to more traditional methods. Considerable doubts are expressed in the educational literature about how frequently this question can be answered in the affirmative, and accompany doubts about the pedagogic approaches used by some of the authors of educational packages using new technologies. [The definition we prefer for pedagogy is 'any conscious activity by one person designed to enhance learning in another'. (Watkins and Mortimore,[5] page 3)] Writing on this subject, Noss and Pachler state that:

all that has happened so far has been the translation into hypermedia of the pedagogic approaches of a previous era. (Noss and Pachler,[6] page 195)

In other words, we haven't necessarily gone forwards in using new technologies in education, and seem in the worst instances to have gone backwards. As we will see later in the chapter, a close analysis of the characteristics of each of the new media available makes it clear that claims such as interactivity within CD-ROM-based packages are seldom true, according to strict learning process criteria.

As learners we are aware of these limitations ourselves, and dissatisfaction about the nature of the learning process when using CD-ROMs is commonplace:

The level of technology isn't all that well developed. They give you a scenario—different pathways, but there's only two or three pathways. It's not the same thing as having a discussion. (Pinder,[2] page 16)

Despite the doubts expressed some progress has clearly been made. We have moved well beyond what Heppell[7] (in Mortimore,[8] page 196) called the initial stage of 'topicality' where the computer was the focus of activity, and the second stage of 'surrogacy' where the computer was viewed as a surrogate teacher, to a third stage (of 'progression') where more sophisticated software on stand-alone computers is used to facilitate problem solving activities. Beyond that we have also moved to the massive potential of the Internet, and software which supports truly interactive learning networks. Some examples of these are given in a later section (see Examples of practical applications of ICT in online CPD).

From the learner's perspective, anxieties about isolation and the use of new technologies are also commonly expressed:

A lot of the benefits of (educational) meetings are meeting with colleagues, mulling over a problem together. Sometimes when you get a difficult problem in the surgery, to be able to go and chew it over with someone... you get a feel for a problem much better when you can talk to someone directly. There's worry that that type of education will go. It's about getting a feel for the problem with face to face interaction you won't get on screen. (Pinder,[2] page 14)

or:

Education in general practice is sharing and social. We're already isolated in general practice. You can go to a lunchtime meeting with a sandwich and a cup of coffee. You might not come away with much information, but it's sharing and supportive. The computer doesn't give you a sandwich and a cup of coffee! I don't see myself going through the CD-Rom model, sitting at home in front of a CD-Rom. (Pinder,[2] page 15)

Research, however, reveals that anxiety about isolation is not always borne out in reality. LeCourt[9] notes, for instance (page 62 citing Hawisher,[10] pages 88–89) that in highly active synchronous and asynchronous internet based discussions between learners and teachers, the learners can be 'more highly involved and participatory than in other forms of classroom interaction', and 'develop a heightened sense of community'.

For the educational processes that are designed for new educational media, the key issue is *whether they aid learning*, and there is clearly a need for rigorous design to ensure that they do. Laurillard[11] (page 94) has outlined an 'empirically-based teaching strategy' which puts forward design criteria against which new media can be measured. She states:

The learning process must be constituted as a dialogue between teacher and student,* operating at the level of descriptions of actions in the world, recognizing the second-order character of academic knowledge,† and having the following characteristics:

- *discursive* (at the level of conceptions): both teacher's and learners' conceptions are accessible to the other and both topic and task goals can be negotiable; learners must be able to act on, generate and receive *extrinsic feedback* on descriptions appropriate to the topic

*The author is writing from a higher education (university) perspective and thus uses the term student. We have replaced this term with the term learner wherever else we have referred to her work, as it is more appropriate for a CPD context.

†Academic knowledge is second order as it is knowledge of *descriptions* of actions in the world rather than first-order knowledge of the actions themselves. This is relevant to ICT and learning, particularly in the non-clinical context or in experiential learning.

goal; the teacher must be able to reflect on the learner's actions and descriptions and adjust their own descriptions to be more meaningful to the learner.[‡]

- *adaptive* (by the teacher): the teacher can use the relationship between their own and the learner's conception to determine the task goals for the continuing dialogue, in the light of the topic goals and previous interactions.
- *interactive* (at the level of actions): the learners can act to achieve the task goal; they should receive meaningful *intrinsic feedback*[¶] on their actions which relates to the nature of the task goal.
- *reflective*: teachers must support the process by which learners link the feedback on their actions to the topic goal, i.e. link experience to descriptions of experience; the pace of the learning process must be controllable by the learners, so that they can take the time needed for reflection when it is appropriate.

Facilitated learning processes and an analysis of educational media

If we accept that the learning process we are examining can be described as a dialogue between 'teacher' and 'learner', then an analysis of the efficacy of new technologies in a teaching and learning setting is best done by

[‡]Extrinsic feedback does not occur within any situation but as an external comment upon it; it is not a 'natural consequence' of the actions of the learner and therefore is not expressed in the 'world' of the action itself.

[¶]With intrinsic feedback, something changes in the system as a result of the actions of the learner—intrinsic feedback is given as a natural consequence of the actions of the learner.

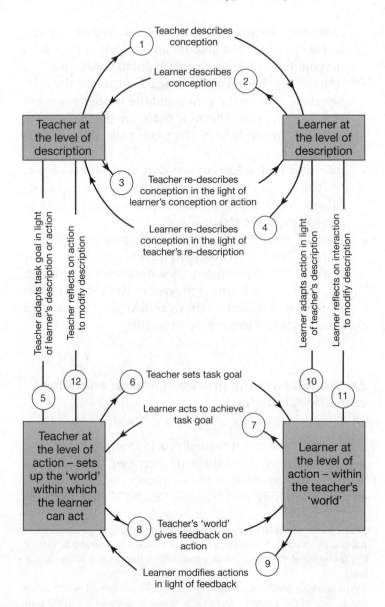

examining what aspects of such a dialogue can be supported by any particular medium. The range of media available will be examined with reference to the 'empirically based teaching strategy' outlined above, and with reference to the diagrammatic analysis of an ideal facilitated learning process in Figure 10.1. For a more detailed discussion of this topic please see Laurillard[11] (pages 100–78).

Audiovisual media

Lecture

This provides a baseline for comparison here. It is neither interactive nor adaptive and does not encourage reflection. Only the teacher is able to communicate their conception. A large burden is placed on the learner in the absence of reflective activity during the lecture and in the absence of any contemporaneous feedback.

Print

This is predominant for logistical rather than pedagogical (teaching process) advantages. Only the teacher is able to communicate their conception. The learner can control the topic focus by re-reading, skipping, browsing, etc., and can control the pace of delivery. Is neither interactive, adaptive, nor reflective. It can be improved somewhat with the inclusion of:

Figure 10.1 Activities necessary to complete a facilitated learning process (adapted from Laurillard,11 page103). In this diagram the complete requirements of a facilitated learning process are represented. The dialogue (or interactivity) between the teacher and the learner is represented in activities 1–4 (at the level of descriptions) and 6–9 (at the level of actions). Adaptation by the teacher and the learner is represented in activities 5–10, and reflection is represented in activities 11 and 12. (Reproduced with kind permission of the publisher.)

- learning objectives
- in-text questions and activities
- references to supplementary texts
- self-assessment questions.

Audio

Audio cassettes are more controllable than lectures but less controllable than print. They lack a visual focus for sighted learners. If combined with visual media (can be text, but could be graphics or preferably three-dimensional objects which can be acted upon by the learner), audio can be truly interactive.

Television

Like the lecture, it is neither discursive, interactive, adaptive, nor reflective, and is not self-paced by the learner. It can use dynamic analogue images as well as language and is very effective in conveying a particular view of the world by 'supplantation' of cognitive processes (Salomon,[12] in Laurillard,[11] page 114) such as, for instance, 'zooming' to a close up supplanting the process of selective attention, or panning from one object to another, 'supplanting' the process of shifting of attention.

Video

Video is adaptive by the learner in contrast to television, but neither fully discursive nor fully interactive. It can be self-paced, thus allowing reflection.

Hypermedia

Hypertext

This is simple to use and teachers can easily create their own courseware. It is not interactive, and is neither adaptive, discursive, nor reflective. Its great strength is controllability by the user but it has little to offer in enabling academic understanding. Hypertext can reduce 'knowledge' to fragments of 'information', the difference being that knowledge is information already transformed such that it is linked in a logical and rhetorical ('expressed in terms calculated to persuade'[13]) way, whereas with information accessible via hyperlinks the link is often merely associative and not logical or rhetorical.

Hypertext systems will be fascinating and motivating for students able to act like researchers in their field, but it will be very easy for them to produce extensively documented rubbish unless the focus is kept firmly on the quality of the knowledge they generate from these systems. (Laurillard,[11] page 126)

Multimedia resources

Commonly a combination of video clips and suchlike linked to text on a CD-ROM, multimedia resources can support 'interactivity' only in the sense of comparing juxtaposed documents. They are neither adaptive nor reflective.

Interactive media

Simulations

The user can make inputs, run the model, and display the results. Non-interactive simulations should be called 'animations ' or 'demonstrations'. Simulations are interactive in that they give intrinsic feedback on the learner's actions. They are not adaptive by the teacher at the task level, and are not discursive or reflective.

Microworlds

They are similar to simulations in that they allow the user to act in a simulated world constrained by limitations imposed by the designer of the world. The difference is that there is a mediating mechanism in the microworld by which the learner can 'act in the world', namely a programming language by means of which they can describe an action, act on the description, and then receive feedback on the action, enabling them to create a re-description and so on. Thus the microworld is interactive, adaptive, and supports reflection.

Modelling

The learner is invited to create their own model of a system, using a mathematical representation of the actions intended, thus manipulating the model itself and not just the parameters within a model as in a microworld.

Adaptive media

Tutorial programs

Tutorial programs and simulations start from the assumption that it is possible for a computer program to emulate a teacher. They should offer as a minimum extrinsic feedback on the action of the learner, and an adaptive task focus related to previous actions and the overall task goal. They frequently use MCQ technique. The risk is that the learner may be able to provide answers to the questions which are not represented in the choices given, thus inviting the learner to 'try to make sense of wrong answers' (Laurillard,[11] page 150). They are adaptive in that the learner's performance governs the task to be set next. Ideally they should be controllable by the learner with an index of contents available at all times. They can offer extrinsic but not intrinsic feedback on actions.

Tutorial simulation

This is a combination of a tutorial program and a simulation and can offer intrinsic feedback if it contains a model of the task which is set, as well as extrinsic feedback as in the tutorial program described above. A tutorial simulation is complex to design as it requires an understanding not only of the subject matter but of the different ways a learner could conceptualize a model. It can be very powerful, adding adaptivity to the interactive capabilities of simulation and modelling.

Tutoring systems (intelligent tutoring systems—ITS)

These set out to do what a one-to-one tutorial would do if augmented by modelling and simulation components. They start from the separation of three key components, namely domain knowledge, the learner's model, and teaching knowledge/strategy (Hartley,[14] in Laurillard,[11] page 157). They are not yet genuinely discursive but an improvement on the MCQ technique of the tutorial program. They can be highly adaptive in that the information used to generate the next action of the system comes partly from domain knowledge and partly from the 'learner model' built up by the system as interactions progress. The choices regarding the relevance of the information used to generate the next action are made by the inbuilt teaching strategy. The learner model created by the system must contain information on errors to decide on the need for more specific tuition. They should still be controllable by the learner. Design and hardware requirements are considerable. They are the only medium to support genuine reflection on the learning experience just undergone.

Discursive media

Audio-conferencing

This is group discussion by telephone and it has some characteristics of face-to-face groups. Someone is chair or mediator. It is partially discursive, but allows no action within a 'world'. If augmented with audio-graphics (such as a whiteboard-like screen on which participants can draw or write—perhaps on a second telephone/ISDN line), it can allow points of view to be expressed more effectively. If a 'common model' is used (via the screen, for instance) upon which all participants can act and see the results, then this becomes 'computer supported collaborative work'—see below.

Video-conferencing

This is chaired or mediated by the 'teacher'. The degree of learner control over the communication is usually similar to a lecture situation, i.e. not that great. As this is a presentational medium as well as a discursive one, the potential level of interaction between teacher and learner which could in theory occur rarely occurs.

Computer-mediated conferencing

This is asynchronous teleconferencing, similar to e-mail. It is somewhat like a normal conference discussion over a longer time span. Responses can be pondered over, topics can be negotiated, and several topics pursued at once. Learner control is relatively high and does allow the learner to 'redescribe their conception in the light of the teacher's redescription' (see Figure 10.1, step 4). It is more fully discursive than the synchronous conferencing media. The success of this medium depends entirely on the fruitfulness of the dialogue generated, and the role of the moderator (who could be a learner and not the teacher) is crucial. The moderator must negotiate goals and timelines for the conference, set up new branches and topics as the discussion progresses, nurture group collaborative processes, and ensure that adequate responses and reactions are given to all relevant contributions.

Computer-supported collaborative work

This is based on interaction between learners in the pursuit of a task. It is not discursive or interactive with the 'teacher', and can break down if the interaction is unsuccessful, but powerful in tandem with adaptive media.

Summary

The close analysis of educational media in this section is important for anyone intent on designing, learning, or using new technologies (see Table 10.1). It is even more important for us as learners to be able to make a discerning choice about what medium we choose to use for our learning. Ideally we should be able to understand in advance whether or not the claims made for the medium are accurate, and the aims, objectives, and outcomes stated achievable.

IM&T and CPD in the clinical environment

Use of clinical information systems in primary care is now widespread with, it is estimated at the time of writing, more than 80% of practices making some use of clinical systems. This section discusses some of the issues surrounding education and training for the use of these systems and for the use of other IM&T resources in the clinical environment.

There is wide variation between practices in the use of IM&T, ranging from those practices that may possess a computer system but make virtually no use of it whatsoever, to those that are paperless or semi-paperless. Use of IM&T in practices can take many forms but it can be broadly summarized under the following headings:

Table 10.1 Media comparison chart

	Print	Audiovision	Television	Video	Self-assessment questionnaires	Hypertext	Multimedia resources	Simulation	Microworlds	Modelling	Tutorial program	Tutoring system	Tutorial simulation	Audioconferencing	Videoconferencing	Computer conferencing	Computer supported collaborative work
Teacher can describe conception	✓	✓	✓	✓	○	✓	✓	○	○	○	✓	✓	✓	✓	✓	✓	○
Learner can describe conception	○	✓	○	○	✓	✓	✓	○	✓	✓	✓	✓	✓	✓	✓	✓	✓
Teacher can re-describe in light of learner's conception or action	○	○	○	○	○	○	○	○	○	○	✓	✓	✓	✓	✓	✓	○
Learner can re-describe in light of teacher's re-description or learner's action	○	✓	○	○	✓	✓	✓	○	○	○	✓	✓	✓	○	○	✓	○
Teacher can adapt task goal in light of	○	○	○	○	○	○	○	○	○	○	✓	✓	✓	○	○	○	○

Statement	C1	C2	C3	C4	C5	C6	C7	C8	C9	C10	C11	C12
Teacher can set task goal	✓	o	o	o	✓	✓	✓	✓	o	✓	✓	o
Learner can act to achieve task goal	✓	o	o	o	✓	✓	✓	✓	o	✓	o	✓
Teacher can set up world to give intrinsic feedback on actions	✓	o	o	o	✓	o	o	✓	o	✓	✓	o
Learner can modify action in light of intrinsic feedback on action	✓	o	o	o	✓	o	o	✓	o	✓	o	o
Learner can adapt actions in light of Teacher's description or learner's re-description	✓	o	o	o	✓	✓	✓	o	o	✓	o	o
Learner can reflect on interaction to modify description	✓	o	o	o	✓	✓	o	o	o	✓	o	o
Teacher can reflect on learner's action to modify re-description	o	o	o	o	✓	o	o	o	o	o	o	o

Adapted from Laurillard,11 page 177.

- uses related to the practice clinical system: patient registration, registration links, item of service links, medical history, consultations, templates/protocols, referrals, prescribing, clinical links, audit and searching, knowledge systems such as Prodigy;
- uses related to standard business software: word processing, spreadsheets, e-mail, Internet, Intranets;
- other clinical uses: NHSNet (information, electronic textbooks, distance learning, e-mail).

Education and training in the use of practice clinical systems

Motivating factors for practices and individual practice members to undertake education and training in the more effective use of clinical systems can be personal, related to the needs of the practice, or a reaction to external requirements such as local clinical governance arrangements. It is relevant to note that the cost of IM&T education and training in general practice is, in most cases, not met by individual practices, but rather by organizations such as health authorities, locally based and variously funded educational organizations, and, more recently, primary care groups (PCGs) or trusts (PCTs). This is in contrast to some other forms of education and training in which the practice team participate, in that in those cases a significant number of practices will self-fund educational activities focused on, say, diabetes management.

There are a number of possible explanations for this, the most likely being:

- there is an increasing abundance of centrally funded IM&T training resources driven by government initiatives such as *Information for Health*[15] and *The NHS Plan*[16] and the desire of PCGs/PCTs to act on their health improvement plans and local implementation strategies.

- IM&T education and training is often perceived by practices to have a lower priority than other types of educational activity targeted at specific clinical areas.

Professional groups in general practice, and attitudes to IM&T education and training

There is an observable variation in the levels of enthusiasm for, and engagement in, education and training for the use of IM&T between different professional groups.

GPs

GPs face severe constraints on their time and it is often this factor that forms a barrier to the increased use of clinical systems by this group. Additionally, although the benefits of using clinical systems in consultations are now unarguable, it is more difficult to show specific overall benefits for the GP personally, as these take some time to filter through. GPs need to be persuaded that good structured consistent clinical records do lead to more efficient care, both in terms of individual patient records and for audit/ development purposes. They also need reassurance that using computers, particularly in the consultation, will not destroy the dynamics of the doctor–patient relationship.

Nurses

Nurses in general are somewhat less resistant to the use of IM&T, particularly where it can be shown that rapid benefit can be found in terms of carrying out routine audits. It is also our experience that it is generally easier to persuade a group of nurses to conform to a particular system for entering data, i.e. all using the same Read Codes* for the same item, than it is to persuade a group of

*Read Codes are: 'a comprehensive list of terms intended for use by all health-care professionals to describe the care and treatment of their

GPs. On the other hand, nurses tend to be reluctant to give up additional means of recording data. A significant number of nurses in our experience not only enter data on the system and in the manual records (which is understandable in some circumstances) but additionally use some form of card index system to record data on specific conditions.

Practice non-clinical staff

Practice non-clinical staff are often the easiest group to persuade of the benefits of IM&T. This is not surprising as it is easier to show clear benefits with administrative tasks, although benefits vary widely with different tasks. Whereas most non-clinical staff would be convinced of the efficiency of a computerized repeat prescription and electronic 'item of service' claims system, few are entirely convinced by appointments systems that fail to perform as flexibly as paper-based systems.

Educational methods

In education and training for IM&T skills, the most effective educational methods are those which are both outcome led and 'hands on'. Table 10.2 summarizes the various types of externally facilitated educational activity available to practice teams.

As well as externally facilitated education and training, much useful educational activity in IM&T skills is organized on a peer-to-peer basis (GP–GP, for example), or tutorial basis (GP–GP Registrar). This type of educational

patients. They enable the capture and retrieval of patient-centred information in natural clinical language within computer systems.' For more information, consult: http://www.cams.co.uk/readcode.html or http://www.coding,nhsia.hns.uk/clinterm/readcodes.asp.

activity is often very practical and effective as it fulfils current, often pressing, need.

Consider the situation where a new GP Registrar starts at a practice which no longer uses manual notes. Although the GP Registrar may be very competent clinically, they are effectively helpless if they do not know how to record information effectively onto the clinical system. A tutorial with the trainer is probably the most effective educational solution in this case.

Similarly, where externally facilitated educational provision is not available or is impractical, there is much value in GPs (and other team members) helping their colleagues (in their own practice and in other practices) to make better use of information systems. The major disadvantage to this approach, however, is the situation where the 'teacher' is not, in fact, using the system effectively, and is therefore merely propagating misinformation.

Individual educational sessions on a one-to-one basis with a professional 'teacher' are perhaps the ideal form of educational activity for learning about the use of IM&T. The sessions can be biased to the learner's needs as well as highly focused. However, this type of educational activity is normally both expensive and relatively inefficient, owing to the problems related to organizing meetings, and should normally, in our view, only form a part, and not all, of an educational programme.

Education and training in IM&T can be an effective vehicle for the development of general medical knowledge and skills in two specific ways:

- the use of knowledge systems within clinical software;
- the use of IM&T in audit—particularly audit of process.

Table 10.2 Some methods of delivering externally facilitated IM&T education and training to GP practices

Method	Target learners	Advantages	Disadvantages
(a) Traditional lecture style talks, normally at a Postgraduate Centre or similar	Mostly GPs but also nurses and sometimes practice managers	Minimum cost per participant	May only be there out of habit and to receive PGEA Points. Potentially little active participation
(b1) 'Hands on' exercise-driven workshops for practice teams (outside the practice)	Whole practice team or selected members	Active participation helps reinforce teaching. Can be relevant and topical	Pointless if not done on practice's clinical system. Notwithstanding above lack of access to 'real' data can be a barrier. Variation in skills or aptitude means danger of boredom and/or confusion for some participants
(b2) 'Hands on' exercise-driven workshops for GPs	GPs	As (b1), and can initiate clinicians discussing or sharing consultation data entry behaviour. Effective if ALL GP team members participate. Potential for all GPs in a PCT to enter data in the same way	As (b1). Time constraints on GPs to travel to external training facility. Costly—particularly if need locum cover. May not be relevant

Method	Target group	Advantages	Disadvantages
(b3) 'Hands on' exercise-driven workshops for nurses	Nurses	As (b1). Effective method of developing templating skills, etc.	As (b1), (b2)
(b4) 'Hands on' exercise-driven workshops for practice managers, etc.	Practice managers or senior admin staff, computing staff	Particularly effective for Searching/Auditing data and strategic use of systems	As (b1)
(b5) 'Hands on' exercise-driven workshops for Practice staff	Any group, i.e. receptionists	Can be very specific, i.e. use of appointment systems	As (b1). Reluctance of participants to travel from the practice
(c1) Practice-based education for whole practice team	Entire practice team	Develops team approach to use of IT	Generally impractical and ineffective except in small practices. Costly
(c2) Practice-based education for selected members of whole practice team	Selected team members but multidisciplinary	As (c1). Can be focused and relevant to practice needs. Long-standing issues can be resolved. Convenient—in practice	Hierarchy problems. GPs may be unwilling to show lack of knowledge in front of other team members. Costly

Table 10.2 *(continued)*

Method	Target learners	Advantages	Disadvantages
(c3) Practice-based education for GPs	GPs only problems	Safe environment to discuss and appropriate educational solutions. Can be relevant and appropriate	GPs sometimes unwilling to display lack of knowledge in front of peers. Individuals may not attend for practical or personal reasons, rendering process less valuable. Lack of time for personal study or reinforcement can reduce value. Costly. Interruptions degrading process more likely in practice
(c4) Practice-based education for nurses	Nurses only	Very focused task-led educational approach can be followed	Interruptions/demands for nurse attention to attend to problems/patients
(c5) Practice-based education for practice managers/computer operators	Computer-using admin staff	As (c4)	New methods can be overruled/sabotaged by GPs/others

Knowledge systems within clinical software

There are a number of knowledge systems available, within clinical software packages, which provide the clinician with immediately available guidance on evidence-based practice. Two examples of these follow.

Drug interaction and contraindication systems

These data-based systems are able to interact with the electronic clinical record. They provide information and warnings if drugs are contraindicated by a recorded patient condition or if an interaction with a previously prescribed drug may occur. Although GPs may be fully aware of most common interactions and contraindications, these systems can protect both the GP and the patient from human error. Additionally, the systems have a secondary educational role in the reinforcement of information regarding interactions and contraindications. Other information such as that for dosage ranges is of use in the same way. A major disadvantage to these prompts is that GPs can find the level of warnings too sensitive and thus can tend to ignore all warnings if they have become too intrusive, although depending on the system the level of sensitivity regarding the display of warnings is often user-configurable.

Prodigy

This is a system available within an increasing number of clinical systems. The way it works varies depending on the clinical system in use, but effectively the user is led towards particular evidence-based guidelines which, in addition to providing prescribing information, may also offer other background information for the GP and patient information. In most cases the guideline is triggered by the entry of a particular Read Code. As well as the practical advantage of using such systems in terms of consistent evidence-based patient care, there is also a significant educational aspect to such systems. Each time the Prodigy guideline is run the user is effectively refreshing their specific knowledge of the subject. Implementations of the Prodigy system vary but most practitioners report finding such extensions to their clinical systems both useful and effective.

Use of IM&T in audit—particularly audit of process

The storing of comprehensive data sets is facilitated in primary care by the supply or construction of templates/protocols relevant to a particular clinical situation. These not only make the process of Read Code selection easier but also act as a set of prompts to remind the user to carry out certain actions and record the results.

It is well recognized that medical audit is one of the key tools for improving the quality of patient care, and clearly the use of computers can make the audit process much more effective. As audit, particularly audit of process, is essentially an educational activity, the effective use of IM&T for audit contributes to a positive educational outcome for the individual practitioner and the team. There are many ways, however, in which audit using computers to search for data can be frustrating and inconclusive, but this is normally due to poor data quality or an inefficient computer system (or both!).

In summary the use of effective clinical IM&T systems has an enormous impact on the global educational boundaries of all members of the primary health care team but the benefits fail to accrue if the education and training related to the use of the clinical system is ineffective in the first instance.

Conclusion

In a workplace setting GPs are in communication with others constantly, their patients, their colleagues, and others in primary care or elsewhere, and their learning experiences from the workplace largely arise from those interactions. In organized learning experiences, whether face to face or mediated by new technologies, we have emphasized the importance of human interaction and feedback for the learner. Designers of educational processes which involve new technologies must always bear the importance of such interaction and feedback in mind, so that false claims are not made for the technologies alone, thus detracting from their real usefulness either as adjuncts to, or as tools for, human communication.

Some relevant websites

- Catchword—online journal search database: more than 900 journals including many on new technologies: http://pinkerton.bham.ac.uk.
- Centre for Health Informatics and Multiprofessional Education: http://www.chime.ucl.ac.uk/.
- Gateway to Health Informatics for Teaching: http://www.chime.ucl.ac.uk/GHIFT/.
- Institute of Educational Technology at the Open University: http://iet.open.ac.uk/.
- International Centre for Distance Learning at the Open University—this site has a wealth of information on all distance learning courses worldwide: http://www-icdl.open.ac.uk/.
- Learning and Teaching Support Network for Medicine, Dentistry and Veterinary Medicine—one of 24

subject centres in the new UK-wide learning and teaching support network (LTSN): http://www.ltsn-01.ac.uk.

• National Electronic Library for Health (NeLH). This is in a pilot stage at time of writing and it is intended that its role will be to provide health care professionals and the public with knowledge and know-how to support health-care-related decisions: http://www.nelh.nhs. uk/.

• NHS Education and Training Programme in Information Management and Technology for Clinicians: http://www.ihcd.org.uk/IMT/imtmain.html.

• North Thames Library and Information Services—links to online medical journals and many Internet-based database resources including online medical dictionaries: http://www.nthames-health.tpmde.ac.uk/ rliulishome.html.

Examples of practical applications of ICT in online CPD

A web-based MSc in Primary Care is offered by the Department of Primary Care and Population Sciences, University College London (http://www.ucl.ac.uk/prim-care-popsci/msc/index.html) which uses software called WebCT (Web Course Tools—available at http://www. webct.com/). This course offers the possibility of synchronous and asynchronous computer conferencing with particular emphasis on the importance of interactivity in the learning process.

In North Thames East, Respiratory Specialist Registrars in-hospital training posts belong to an online virtual community called the 'Specialist Registrar internet training environment' (SpRite—http://194.83.41.144/) which uses FirstClass software (available at http://www.softarc.com/), and has been running since 1996. This provides tutorials and assessments which include x-rays and other images, the capacity for secure individual tutor and student communication, and also synchronous and asynchronous discussion between students. It has now expanded to provide ChestNet (http://www.chestnet.net/), a resource on chest medicine for the whole medical community, and hopes to develop European links.

The Computerised Obstetrics and Gynaecology Automated Learning Analysis (KOALA)[17] is a multicentred Internet-based learning portfolio which allows residents in a Canadian program to record patient encounters and to document critical incidents or elements of surprise during the encounters. By prompting the student to reflect on these learning experiences, the program encourages residents to articulate questions which can be directly pursued through hypertext links to evidence-based literature (http://www.uottawa.ca/academic/med/obgyn/promot. html).

The WISDOM project[18] applies Internet technologies to create a virtual classroom in health informatics for primary care professionals. Participants use a facilitated e-mail discussion list supported by a website which provides online resources and an archive of teaching materials (http://wisdomnet.inetc.net/index.html).

References

1. Rennison AJ. *Essential Guide to Primary Care Computing, a Practice Guide.* Reading: Petroc Press, 1999.
2. Pinder R. GPs and their current use of IT in addressing their educational needs: an old debate in new clothing? *Report for Thames*

Postgraduate Medical & Dental Education North Thames (East) GP Department. Unpublished ms. Brunel University: Centre for the Study of Health, 2000.

3. Angood, P. B., (1999). Critical Care Telemedicine: a Toy or a Tool? *New Horizons* 1999; **7**: 229–35.

4. Chambers M. The efficacy and ethics of using digital multimedia for educational purposes. In: Tait A, Mills R, eds. *The Convergence of Distance and Conventional Education.* London: Routledge, 1999.

5. Watkins C, Mortimore P. Pedagogy: What do we know? In: Mortimore P, ed. *Understanding Pedagogy and its Impact on Learning.* London: Sage, 1999.

6. Noss R, Pachler N. The challenge of new technologies: doing old things in a new way, or doing new things? In Mortimore P, ed. *Understanding Pedagogy and its Impact on Learning.* London: Sage, 1999.

7. Heppell S. Teacher education, learning and the information generation: the progression and evolution of educational computing against a background of change. *Journal of Information Technology for Teacher Education* 1993; 2(2): 229–37.

8. Mortimore P, ed. *Understanding Pedagogy and its Impact on Learning.* London, Sage, 1999.

9. LeCourt D. The ideological consequences of technology and education; the case for critical pedagogy. In: Selinger M, Pearson J, eds. *Telematics in Education.* Oxford: Pergamon, 1999.

10. Hawisher GE. Electronic meetings of the minds: research, electronic conferences, and composition studies. In: Hawisher GE, LeBlanc P, eds. *Re-imagining Computers and Composition: Teaching and Research in the Virtual Age* Portsmouth, New Hampshire: Heinemann-Boynton/Cook, 1992.

11. Laurillard D. *Rethinking University Teaching.* London: Routledge, 1993.

12. Salomon G. *Interaction of Media, Cognition and Learning.* San Francisco: Jossey-Bass, 1979.

13. Ryan S, ed. *Oxford English Dictionary,* CD edn. Oxford: Oxford University Press, 1999.

14. Hartley JR. The design and evaluation of an adaptive teaching system. *International Journal of Man-Machine Studies* 1973; **5**(3): 421–36.

15. Department of Health UK. *Information for Health: An information Strategy for the Modern NHS.* London: HMSO, 1998. http://www.doh.gov.uk/farend/index.html.

16. Department of Health. *The NHS Plan.* London: The Stationery Office, 2000. http://www.nhs.uk/nationalplan/default.html.

17. Fung MFK, Walker M, Fung KFK, *et al.* An Internet-based learning portfolio in resident education: the KOALA™ multicentre programme. *Medical Education* 2000; **34**: 474–9.

18. Fox NJ, Dolman EA, Lane P, O'Rourke AJ, Roberts C. The WISDOM Project: training primary care professionals in informatics in a collaborative 'virtual classroom'. *Medical Education* 1999; **33**: 365–70.

Further reading

The following books are recommended for their analyses of the issues surrounding the use of new technology in educational settings.

Kommers P, Grabinger S, Dunlap J, eds. *Hypermedia Learning Environments—Instructional Design and Integration*. Mahwah, NJ: Laurence Erlbaum, 1996. ISBN 0805818294.

Laurillard D. *Rethinking University Teaching*. London: Routledge, 1993. ISBN 0415092892.

Selinger M, Pearson J, eds. *Telematics in Education - Trends and Issues*. Oxford: Pergamon, 1999. ISBN 008042788X.

Tait A, Mills R, eds. *The Convergence of Distance and Conventional Education*. London: Routledge, 1999. ISBN 0415194288.

11 Learning from patients

PATRICIA WILKIE

Introduction

Every patient provides two questions—what can be learnt from the patient and secondly what can be done for him.[1]

Formal scientific medical education began in the eighteenth century in the autopsy room. Students examined the cadaver. Neither the deceased not their relatives were likely to have consented or been actively involved in this educational process. By the beginning of the twentieth century, changes had already taken place. Carl Binger (1889–1976) describes these changes:[2]

... a shift in emphasis has already happened ... from post mortem to laboratory to clinic. No longer were anatomists content with describing bones, muscles and nerves, or pathologists with describing the gross and microscopic appearance of tissue. Insight and understanding of mechanisms and processes had become increasingly important.

The importance of the emphasis on scientific medicine was described by Daniel Cathell (1839–1925):[3]

Working with the microscope and making analysis of the urine, sputum, blood and other body fluids as an aid to diagnosis, will not only bring fees and lead to valuable information regarding your patient's condition, but will also give you reputation and professional respect, by investing you in the eyes of the public, with the benefits of being a very scientific man.

The patient will still not have played an active part in this phase of medical education. Samples of fluid or tissue will have been given or taken during surgical or other procedures. The real involvement of the patient was not required. The way that modern scientific medicine has developed has not required the active cooperation, involvement, or participation of the patient. The patient's views were not important.

However, the importance for patients of the scientific training of doctors cannot be underestimated. Patients now expect doctors to be familiar with the latest diagnostic tests as well as new and proven treatments. The twentieth century has also witnessed a very considerable change in the pattern of illnesses seen by general practitioners. In his *Manual of General Medical Practice*, the Leeds general practitioner W Stanley Sykes (1894–1960) cited influenza as the commonest complaint seen in his practice followed by acute bronchitis, tonsilitis, measles, whooping cough, and other infectious diseases.[4] Sykes had more patients with pneumonia than with cancer and more than half his patients with pneumonia died. It is well known that the disease picture changed dramatically in the twentieth century. Improved living standards, better nutrition, and effective drug and immunization therapies have meant a decline in acute infectious diseases. These have been replaced by cancer, coronary heart disease, strokes, mental health problems, Alzheimer's disease, and other chronic diseases. As Porter says:[5] 'The age of acute illness has yielded to the age of chronic disease.' Thus at the beginning of the twenty-first century, very many patients have had to learn to live with chronic and degenerative diseases. The causes of many of these illnesses remains unknown and it is not yet possible to prevent or cure them. To find out more about these illnesses, it is necessary to listen to those who have them.

The rise of patient organizations

The 1960s saw the development of the critical consumer able to question established traditions and establishment of many health-related organizations such as the National Childbirth Trust (NCT), and the National Association for Women and Children in Hospital (NAWCH) to press for the introduction of change.[6] These organizations demonstrated that what seemed obvious to patients and users of services did not seem so readily understood by professionals. The NCT campaigned for continuity of care for women during pregnancy and for choice in the place of confinement. Williamson[7] describes how parents, convinced of the importance of the need for children in hospital to have regular and continuing contact with their parents, pressurized through NAWCH for the universal adoption of unrestricted visiting, for the provision of accommodation to enable mothers to stay in hospital with their child, and for better play facilities in children's wards. More general organizations concerned with health, including the Patients Association and community health councils in England and Wales and local health councils in Scotland, also emerged during this period The importance of all these organizations is that they give information to the public about health services and their availability. They also give information to patients and their relatives about what to expect in different illnesses and what treatments are available. Furthermore, the organizations are able to lobby on behalf of their members.

The first half of the twentieth century, dominated by acute illnesses, was also a period when the doctor–patient relationship was characterized by paternalism and an intrinsic confidence and assurance that 'doctor knows best'.[6] By the second half of the twentieth century, the causes of infectious diseases were at last understood. Immunization programmes were developed and antibiotics were providing effective treatment. But there were no magic bullets for chronic illnesses. It is not surprising, therefore, that the second half of the twentieth century saw a great increase in self-help organizations concerned with chronic illnesses, including those concerned with arthritis, asthma, diabetes, mental illnesses, and multiple sclerosis. In recent years, many of these organizations have grouped together to form 'umbrella' organizations such as the Long-term Medical Conditions Alliance (LMCA), the Genetic Interest Group (GIG), and the Neurological Alliance, for more effective lobbying and for communicating the interests of their members.

The National Association of Patient Participation Groups (NAPP) is the patient organization peculiar to general practice. NAPP was founded in 1978 to:

- give doctors and patients the opportunity to discuss topics of mutual interest in the practice;
- provide a means for patients to make positive suggestions about both the practice and their own health care;
- encourage health education activities within the practice;
- act as representative groups to influence the local provision of health and social care.

In the past, the activities of NAPP have tended to focus on what are described as service activities, including fundraising to improve amenity in the surgery as well as providing sitting services for the housebound and creches in the surgery. Increasingly, however, groups are involved in carrying out surveys of patient views, in the training of staff, and in providing information for patients as well as being represented on practice management committees.

Patients with chronic illnesses are increasingly able to acquire more technical information about their illness from a variety of sources including their own disease association. The recent edition of *Pathways*,[8] the magazine for people affected by multiple sclerosis, has articles on:

- alternative therapies
- benefits
- alternative medicines
- current research into MS
- NICE and interferon.

There is also an informative letter page. Authors who come from the UK and overseas often give e-mail addresses, allowing for a much wider and ready exchange of information than has hitherto been possible. Disease organizations also can offer to patients the most up-to-date information about treatments available, as well as information about major research being carried out. These organizations enable members to become more informed patients, to help themselves, and to give them confidence.

Health-related voluntary organizations continue to develop, established by members often to highlight new problems. Organizations such as the National Association for Child Organ Retention (NACOR), Stolen Hearts, and the Bristol Heart Children's Action Group were all established in the last three years to support parents, highlight issues resulting from the Bristol Royal Infirmary Inquiry (2000) and to recommend change resulting from parents' concerns about the retention of tissue following post-mortem examination. Voluntary health organizations give support to their members but are also able to influence government and practitioners working with patients.

Involving the expert patient

The increasing number of people with chronic illness, the failure of modern medicine to cure, concerns by governments about the increasing costs of treatments, and the mounting evidence of a lack of compliance by patients in treatment regimens have all served as an impetus for the promotion of involving the patient in their health care.[9] However, the concept of patient participation in their health care was embodied in the 1978 WHO Alma-Ata Declaration.[10] Many of the early studies involving patient participation in their health care have focused on secondary care.[11] Conditions such as hypertension, which are mainly managed in general practice, lend themselves to greater involvement of the patient in their own care. This is so obvious, as once on medication the patient is largely self-monitoring. The patient is also likely to choose a treatment regimen that suits their lifestyle.[12]

A small study by Simms[13] examined the management of blood pressure from the patient perspective and assessed the views of the patients about their involvement in the management of their hypertension. The majority of patients in this study were relatively knowledgeable about blood pressure control and lifestyle changes that may be needed. The author suggests that patients with hypertension, and particularly those with newly diagnosed hypertension, would benefit from participation in the management of their condition. What is interesting is that the patients in this study perceived the management of their condition as something that was done to them by doctors and other health-care professionals. Cahill[14] suggests that to enable patients to participate in the management of their condition there is a need to narrow the knowledge gap between patients and doctors. The assumption here is that patients need to learn more and health-care professionals need to communicate better. Indeed, patients may need to be helped to understand that they do have the expertise and can take more responsibility for their own care. But the knowledge gap between health-care professionals and patients must also include information about the patient perspective for the professionals.

The provision of care in general practice for patients with asthma has changed as a result of the 1993 chronic disease management contract,[15,16] which introduced a standardized package of care in the form of asthma clinics that patients would attend on a regular basis and which are audited by health authorities using process criteria. Previously, patients had been looked after on an individual basis. There is evidence that as many as one-third of people in the community with asthma have a high morbidity from their asthma.[17] A recent study by Paterson and Britten[18] examined the views of general practice patients with asthma. The facilities valued by patients included:

- to be able to consult a 'professional' quickly when the need arises either by telephone or by attending the surgery;
- to be given regular support and monitoring;
- to receive accessible care from a health professional with whom they have developed a relationship;
- to have expert asthma care at home when housebound;
- to have a choice of appointment times to fit in with other commitments;
- to have acknowledgement of their own self-knowledge about their own or their child's illness;
- to have access to expert professional advice about medication.

Paterson and Britten suggest that in order for asthma care to be useful to patients and for patients to make the best use of the care available it needs to be provided in a way that allows individual choice and freedom. That is certainly true. But what this research also demonstrates is the importance of seeking the views of patients, and, in particular, to seek the views of relevant patients before major changes to services that affect patients are introduced.

In 1999, following the publication of the white paper *Saving Lives: Our Healthier Nation,* the government announced the establishment of the Expert Patient Task Force (EPTF). One of the first tasks of the EPTF was to design a programme to address the needs of people in England living with a chronic disease. An outcome of the EPTF is to develop programmes of lay-led self-management for people with chronic conditions. Patients themselves, the experts, lead these programmes and show how they work, to both other patients and professionals. As the chief Medical Officer, Professor Liam Donaldson, said at a conference 'Designing an Expert Patient Programme', 11 July 2000:

The concepts of self-management and the expert patient offer the potential to do something unusual. This is a paradigm shift to put patients in the driving seat. . . .

One of the first of the self-management programmes is that developed in the USA by Kate Lorig to help people cope with arthritis and fibromyalgia[19] and now followed by many patients in other countries. The programmes began in 1979 to help people with arthritis change their activities and abilities, decrease their pain, and, most importantly, develop confidence in themselves as caretakers for their own bodies. This programme was developed by people with arthritis and the programmes are led by patients. Furthermore, the programmes are not intended to replace medical care or the need for people to consult doctors. They provide a supplement to medical care and enable patients to develop control over their life with a chronic illness.

Organization of care

Patients have a whole wealth of personal experience of how the range of health and social services work and link together. It is foolhardy not to listen to such expert witnesses.[20] In 1988, the Picker Institute at Harvard Medical School developed a programme of organizational learning driven by and based on the priorities of patients. In 1999, Lothian University Hospitals Trust embarked on a study based on the work of Picker Institute. Patients were directly involved in the development of questionnaires. Former patients, including adults, children, parents, and new mothers, met with independent researchers individually or in focus groups to talk freely about what mattered to them while they were in hospital. Their emphasis was very clearly on matters of clinical care, communication, coordination of care, information, and education.[21] As a result, the questionnaires asked patients about issues concerning clinical care and treatment. This is in contrast with many patient satisfaction surveys, which tend to focus on topics concerning amenity. The first part of this on-going survey in Edinburgh reported in May 2000. Whilst this is a study based on the experiences of patients recently discharged from hospital, there were particular aspects that have implications for general practice. For example, women using maternity services were unhappy and felt that they were left in limbo by a policy which stated that they would not be informed of test results when the results were negative. This is an interesting finding as not informing patients of negative test results is a common policy for many screening and test procedures carried out in both hospital and in the community.

Researchers also found that patients became extremely anxious or frustrated when staff contradicted each other. This indicated to patients that staff did not appear to know what they were doing and points to the need for doctors and other practice staff to be able, where appropriate, to give consistent information to patients.

The views of patients can be used to identify areas of patient needs and to influence policy. A project, 'Patients Influencing Purchasers' by the LMCA involved patients with chronic illnesses working with health authorities to set standards. In addition, the LMCA collected the views of many people with long-term medical conditions through questionnaires, telephone interviews, group discussions, and interviews . The essence of the findings of these projects were:

• people need to be treated as people, not labelled as patients;
• the expertise of individuals and their organizations should be used;
• services should be set in the context of achieving greater social inclusion for people with long-term medical conditions.

The recommendations in their report[22] were focused on the National Health Service Executive, health authorities, trusts, and voluntary organizations.

Patients can also be involved in the development of clinical guidelines. The Scottish Intercollegiate Guidelines Network (SIGN), widely used by Scottish general practitioners, involves lay people on their working groups.

Involvement of consumers in research

It is now increasingly accepted that the outcome in certain aspects of the medical care of individual patients is likely to be more successful if the patient is more involved in the decisions about their treatment. If research reflects the needs and views of consumers, it is more likely to produce results that can be used to improve practice. Furthermore, the involvement of consumers and patients in the research process is likely to lead to research that is more relevant and likely to be used.[23]

There are different ways in which patients and consumers can be involved in the whole process of research. Involving patients in the research process can:

- help to ensure that issues important to patients are identified;
- help to ensure that research does not measure only outcomes that are identified and considered as important by the professionals;
- help to ensure that technologies that are developed are acceptable to patients;
- help with recruitment;
- help to include otherwise marginalized groups to contribute to research;
- help in the dissemination of results;
- help to ensure that changes resulting from research are implemented.

(The above list is adapted from *Guidelines for Grant Applicants Involving Consumers in Research* and is produced by the Consumers in NHS Research Support Unit, 1999.)

Not only do researchers need to ensure that research does not exploit its subjects, but they also need to consider how the research could improve the lives of those being researched. The best way to achieve this is to work in partnership with users and research subjects. Users can help to improve the design of research and encourage recruitment and compliance, if they feel it is worthwhile. Research will then be of better quality and more relevant to the experiences of patients and carers.[23] In some situations, patients can also help decide the topics that should be researched as well as areas that should be audited as the services in the future may be influenced by both research and audit. Medical research, including social and psychological research into the effects of different treatments, is vitally important for both the present and future generations. The person that should be involved in the research process is the subject of the research. Subjects may be:

- individual patients
- groups of patients
- parents, relatives or carers
- consumer groups and patient organizations
- users of the services.

Patients cannot make informed choices about treatment without knowing about the likely success and side-effects of different treatments as well as what is likely to happen if they have no treatment at all. The criteria chosen to assess the effectiveness of treatments are therefore very important. Patients as well as professionals can define what factors are measured as outcomes for treatments. Patients can also comment on existing outcome measures. For example, length of survival is the traditional measure of success for many treatments, but this does not take account of the quality of the remaining life. Patients, carers and professionals may have different views of what is a good outcome of treatment and assess the quality of life after treatment differently.[24] Medical research has often ignored the patients' experiences of the treatment, preferring to measure physiological changes. Researchers may have to consider ways of using qualitative methodologies in order to capture the patients' perspective.

In some areas, participatory research is possible and, in fact, the best way of getting the information wanted. The great benefit of participatory research is that it can be of real benefit to those who participate. They can gain new skills and confidence. For example, mental health service users can be trained to interview other mental health service users, or people from self-help groups. Assessing the needs of particular communities has been successfully undertaken by directly involving local people who can be interviewers. In certain circumstances, local people may be the only people who would be acceptable to their community and who could obtain information from a community who view outsiders with suspicion. The health needs of travellers may be neglected. The views of 'new age' travellers concerning the transmission of HIV and their views on general health awareness were successfully investigated by a team of new age travellers with support from voluntary sector workers and academics.[25] Researchers can learn from the involvement of the patient or subject in the whole research process. Such involvement can also help improve the quality of the research.

Interprofessional education

In 1987, the Centre for the Advancement of Inter-Professional Education (CAIPE) was established to facilitate the development of interprofessional education. The complexity of patient care both in hospitals and in the community nearly always requires the involvement of a number of agencies and professions. Collaboration between professions is now a key aspect in the delivery of health care as well as in the planning of workforces and in staff development. CAIPE believes that to make the best use of all the skills of the different professional groups does require considerable trust and understanding amongst those involved and the best way of encouraging and developing this is by interprofessional edcucation at all levels, including pre-qualification, post-qualification, and continuing education. An aspect of interprofessional education must be that it should now include, wherever possible, the patient and/or carer as part of the team and this is increasingly recognized by CAIPE.[26]

Took and Bell[27] involved users of mental health services and carers in post-qualifying interprofessional education. The research found that both service users and carers were very willing to be involved in education. The research also found that students welcomed the involvement of users and carers. The authors suggest that service users and carers have much to offer providers of education through their experience of mental illness and mental health services and that this is a resource that may not be available from anywhere else. They also have a valuable part to play in the development of curricula, the delivery of training, the evaluation of courses, as well as involvement in student research projects. It is important to remember that the perspectives of service users and carers are different. Both need to be listened to in equal partnership with health and social care professionals whose views are influenced by the norms and values of their profession and by the policies of the organization that they work for.

Patient involvement in the education of doctors

Patients have always been involved in the education of doctors but as a subject with a particular medical problem to be looked at, prodded, and examined. In these circumstances, the patient is there simply to answer the questions of either the student or those teaching. Alternatively, the student may write up case histories of patients. In both these situations the patient is passive in this educational process. While involving patients in this way may remain a necessary part of the education of doctors, there are ways of involving patients more actively. For example, it is not uncommon for medical students to sit in on a consultation in general practice and then discuss later with the general practitioner their observations of the consultation and what they had learned from it. However, it does not appear routine for the student also to discuss with the patient how useful the consultation had been for them. Such a practice could extend the student's knowledge and awareness of the patient perspective.[28]

Medical students are increasingly spending time early in their degree in community placements. It seems important that whenever possible students are able to spend time with individual patients and families with chronic illness. Expert patients or representatives from patient organizations can be invited to give seminars or individual lectures about the implications of living with particular illnesses.

However, these are 'formal' methods of involving patients in the education of doctors. There is very considerable evidence from doctors that they have always learned from their patients. The importance of listening to patients and to the story of the patient have been extolled for centuries by many doctors. Perhaps this message needs to be reinforced in the education and training of doctors.

Patient involvement in assessment and examination

The medical profession in the UK wishes to retain its privilege of being a self-regulating profession. There are changes. Already one-third of the members of the General Medical Council (GMC), the regulatory authority for the medical profession, are lay members. These lay members are involved in the assessment visits of poorly performing doctors as well as being involved in the process of setting standards. In 1999, the GMC announced that all doctors will be required on a regular basis to demonstrate that they continue to be fit to practise. This process has been termed 'revalidation'. The Royal College of General Practitioners (RCGP) has established a working group to develop the GMC's proposals for general practitioners. There are two lay members from the Patient Liaison Group (PLG) of the RCGP on this working group. Lay people will also be involved in the revalidation process working alongside medical colleagues.[29]

There are situations where patients, lay people, may be part of the examining or assessment team. The RCGP has introduced lay assessors for the senior of the awards of the RCGP, the Fellowship by Assessment (FBA). These lay assessors attend with the two medical colleagues the assessment day for the candidate and play an equal part in the assessment process. Equally importantly, there is lay membership on the working group involved in the development of new criteria. The RCGP also plans to introduce lay assessors to the awards of Membership by Assessment of Performance (MAP) and Quality Practice Award (QPA). The RCGP needs to be congratulated for, to the best of my knowledge, being the first medical Royal College to fully involve lay people in the assessment process of their post-qualification awards. For some years lay people, that is, people who do not have a medical qualification, have been involved in teaching in the undergraduate medical curriculum and as examiners. These are usually social scientists, statisticians, and staff of the university who are different from the lay assessors involved at the RCGP, who are independent people with particular expertise in and knowledge of patient views.

Conclusion

Neither patients nor doctors have a monopoly of wisdom, but each needs to recognise that within the limits of current knowledge, it is the patient who determines what is an acceptable outcome. [Quoted in *The Patient's Network* **1**(2): Autumn 1996]

This book is about education and training in primary care. This chapter is entitled 'Learning from Patients'. Many ways that practitioners can learn from patients have been discussed including:

• listening to the patient in the consultation;
• involving patients in research;
• involving patients in quality initiatives and the development of guidelines;
• accepting that patients have a valuable part to play in assessment of doctors;
• involving patients in interprofessional education;
• involving patients at practice level.

It is understood that in the present health system with shortage of staff and increased demands on the service, the message from this chapter may seem unrealistic. I do not believe that is the case. Listening to patients and involving them as partners is a learning experience and is, in the twenty-first century, essential for the delivery of quality patient care.

References

1. Cushing H. *Consecratio Medici and Other Papers*. Boston: Little, Brown, 1928.
2. Binger C. (1889–1976). Cited in reference 5.
3. Cathell D. (1924) Cited in Starr P. *The Social Transformation of American Medicine*. New York: Basic Books, 1982.
4. Sykes WS. *A Manual of General Medical Practice*. London: HK Lewis,1927.
5. Porter R. *The Greatest Benefit to Mankind: a Medical History of Humanity from Antiquity to the Present*. London: Harper Collins, 1997.
6. Wilkie P. The patient perspective. In: Simms J, ed. *Primary Health Care Sciences*. London: Whurr Publishers, 1999.
7. Williamson C. *Whose Standards? Consumer and Professional Standards in Health Care*. Milton Keynes: Open University Press, 1992.
8. *Pathways* The information magazine for people affected by MS. 2001; **January/February.**
9. Brearley S. *Patient Participation*. London: Scutari, 1990.
10. World Health Organization. *Alma-Ata (1978) Primary Health Care: Report of the International Conference*. Geneva: WHO, 1978.
11. Wennberg JE, Barry MJ, Fowler FJ, Mulley A. Outcomes research, PORTs and health care reforms. *Annals of the New York Academy of Sciences* 1993; **703**: 52–62.
12. Cameron K, Gregor F. Chronic illness and compliance. *Journal of Advanced Nursing* 1987; **12**: 671–6.
13. Simms J. What influences a patient's desire to participate in the management of their hypertension? *Patient Education and Counseling* 1999; **38**(3): 185–94.
14. Cahill J. Patient participation: a concept analysis. *Journal of Advanced Nursing* 1996; **24**: 561–71.
15. Department of Health. FHSL, 3/17. London: DoH, 1993.
16. Department of Health and the Welsh Office. *Statement of Fees and Allowances*. [Paragraph 30, Schedule 3]. London: DoH, 1972.
17. Barritt PW, Staples EB. Measuring success in asthma care: a repeat audit. *Family Practice* 1991; **41**: 232–6.
18. Paterson C, Britten N. Organising primary health care for people with asthma: the patient's perspective. *British Journal of General Practice* 2000; **50**: 299–303.
19. Lorig K, Fries JF. *The Arthritis Handbook: a Tested Self-management Program for Coping with Arthritis and Fibromyalgia*, 4th edn. New York: Adddison-Wesley, 1995.
20. Berwick DM. The total customer relationship in healthcare: broadening the bandwith. *Journal of Quality Improvement* 1997; **23**: 245–50.

21. Straw P, Bruster S, Richards N, Lilley S.J. Sit up, take notice. *Health Service Journal* 2000; **11 May**: (issue no.5704). 24–6.
22. Long Term Medical Conditions Alliance. *Patients Influencing Purchasers.* London: LMCA, 1999.
23. Hogg C. Involving patients in research. In: Carter YH, Shaw S, Thomas C, eds. *Master Classes in Primary Research.* London: Royal College of General Practitioners, 2000.
24. Frater A. Health outcomes: a challenge to the status quo. *Quality in Health Care* 1996; **1**: 87–8.
25. Oliver S, Buchanan P. *Examples of Lay Involvement in Research and Development.* London: Social Science Research Unit, London University Institute of Education, 1997.
26. Tope R. Meeting the challenge: introducing service users and carers into the education equation. *CAIPE Bulletin* 1998; **15**: 11.
27. Took M, Bell L. Voices of experience: users and carers, partners in post-qualifying IPE. *CAIPE Bulletin* 1998; **15**: 12–13.
28. Williamson C, Wilkie P. Editorial: Teaching medical students in general practice: respecting patients' rights. *British Medical Journal* 1997; **315**: 1108–9.
29. Royal College of General Practitioners. *Members Reference Book.* London: RCGP, 2000.

12 Higher degrees: their role in education and training for primary care

AMANDA HOWE

Background

'Higher degrees' are all postgraduate qualifications that involve a substantive piece of original research work: this definition covers Masters (MMedSci, MSc, MPhil) and doctorates (PhD, or MD for those with a previous medical qualification). They range from taught courses to independently completed single theme projects, usually span 1–6 years of study depending on whether full- or part-time, and can be undertaken at any point in one's adult life. Holding such a qualification is regarded as an essential step to an academic career, but also by many as evidence of serious scholarship and intellectual attainment.

Professional training for health care does not seem to have consistent links to the academic culture of research. For example, the summative assessments for vocational accreditation in general practice include skills in critical reading and clinical audit, but not in research skills *per se*. Some registrar level trainings and CME programmes have attempted the development of additional modules which can be accredited towards a Masters degree (H Davies, personal communication), but these are by no means part of a core national training curriculum. While it appears likely that those completing training at a research-oriented medical school will both undertake higher degrees and take up academic careers,[1] the majority of primary care staff will have trained outside such settings and the concept of training for research may sound very alien.

So why should anyone in primary care, with their vocational qualifications already under their busy belts, be willing or keen to engage with such an undertaking? Indeed, would they be capable? Many people working in primary care have not been to 'university' on the conventional 3-year course; even the doctors will not for the most part have done a full undergraduate degree, with its emphasis on generic academic skills and scholarship for its own sake. Higher degrees will be viewed by many colleagues as either mysterious, irrelevant, or too difficult, and it is likely that few in primary care will be drawn to this choice: but you cannot know what you choose or refuse till well informed, so read on and see what you think!

The principles of undertaking a higher degree

Although grouped together by their postgraduate nature, the undertaking of a taught course or a single research study are very different experiences, and this chapter will divide the two for some sections. Their common features include:

- necessary background educational achievement: at minimum an undergraduate degree, a medical or graduate nursing qualification, or evidence of equivalent expertise;
- formal registration with an accredited academic unit. For a taught course this will be the host institution,

even if it is undertaken by distance learning: for MD or PhD, it must be either a current employer or your original university;

- undertaking any taught elements required, and successful completion of necessary assignments;
- deciding on an original research question (one that no-one else appears to have answered);
- reviewing the literature, and refining the question to a level of necessary clarity;
- designing a research study whereby the question could be answered, and deciding appropriate methods to undertake this;
- doing the data collection/field work;
- analysing the results;
- writing and discussing the findings;
- having the work assessed by independent examiners;
- hopefully, being awarded the degree!

Undertaking a higher degree may in many circumstances also result in presenting completed work as conference papers or published articles.

On a taught Masters course, the independent research project, or 'dissertation' as it is more commonly called, will be only one component, and will count for only around one-third of the 'credits' awarded towards the qualification, whereas for MPhil, MD, or PhD the whole qualification is based on a single research question or group of themed studies. The amount of work also varies: PhD is expected to be the most detailed, and therefore to take the longest, whereas a taught Masters might be completed in a year. Table 12.1 shows a full outline.

Table 12.1 Higher degrees—completion periods and levels of
supervision

Type of degree	Completion period	Level of supervision
MA, MSc, MMedSci	1 year full time Increasing number of flexible part time modular courses	Taught course with submission of dissertation
MPhil	1 year full time Usual route to register for Mphil then possibility of upgrading to PhD	Combination of taught course and supervision
MD	2 years full time Most GPs combine MD with clinical work and commonly submit in 3–5 years	Technically an unsupervised degree although a nominal supervisor needs to be recognized for regular guidance
PhD	3 years full time Part-time option less common but may be available	Personal supervisor and often advisory/ reference group identified for further support

Why would you consider doing a higher degree?

Several studies have shown that the vast majority of those
who do a higher degree continue to be active researchers
after they graduated.[2,3] Others have recorded the benefits
to peers through active publication by researchers, and
their uptake of new academic commitments that contribute to service and the development of their disciplines.[4]

Work continues to demonstrate the 'added value' to clinical practice of education,[5] and some have questioned whether the 'cult' of the original research degree is justifiable.[6] However, there is evidence that professional isolation and burnout can be reduced by participation in higher degrees, at least at taught Masters level,[7] and this will be the main motivation for many with a need for mental stimulation in the face of hard daily work, or a wish for some time to look at practice from a more critical and reflective point of view. Other motivators may be personal contacts and role models, suggestions from colleagues or mentors, local opportunities, and a prevailing culture in primary care which seeks to encourage research activity.[8] Anecdotally, there appears to be a link between contact with an academic unit for teaching and an increasing awareness of research opportunities (see case studies later in this chapter). So if you teach health profession students, be very careful—you might get the research bug next!

The practicalities of doing a higher degree

If you start to consider the possibility of doing a higher degree, you will need to consider the following:

- whether you want to do a taught course or a single piece of research on a pet topic;
- whether you want to do this gently over a long period or get on with it full time;
- what is available locally, or whether you can find anything on the Internet that would suit you;
- what is offered by your previous 'parent' university;
- what funding might be available to support you with fees, equipment, and buying your time out of service;

- who else is embarking on a similar adventure, or who is ahead of you on the path.

There are three key resources for obtaining this kind of information: local colleagues already known to you; your local academic departments of general practice/nursing/primary care or similar; and directories that are available either on the Internet or via a national or regional resource centre such as your NHS Regional Office, or the Royal Colleges. Universities usually have a graduate school or similar who will welcome general enquiries, while an academic unit of your own disciplinary background will advise on working up an application or research proposal. Often one local link into primary care will lead to all the others, and some units have a 'one-stop shop' for primary care staff making initial enquiries about research. A list of websites is to be found in Table 12.2.

Table 12.2   Internet resources for information about research and academic centres

http://www.rcgp.org.uk/college/activity/research/ The Royal College of GPs	
http://www.mrc.ac.uk/	Medical Research Council
http://scitsc.wlv.ac.uk/ ukinfo/uk.map.html	Entry site for UK universities
http://www.ex.ac.uk/pgms/ nhse.html	For NHS primary care R & D
http://www.ppptrust.org/	PPP Healthcare Medical Trust
http://www.wellcome.ac.uk/	The Wellcome Trust

All these show useful linked sites.

Getting the education and training for higher degrees

Whatever type of higher degree you decide to undertake, there are several key areas for which you will have to plan: making time available, resourcing your information technology requirements, identifying good training and supervision resources, and dealing with a cultural transition. It is important not to register for any degree before you are ready to start, as you will incur fees and eat into your maximum time allowance for completion. However, you can often start to become acquainted with learning resources and options while making final plans for finances and settling on your research question. Most university units will offer some core modules to assist in getting to grips with the library, online resources, and suitable software for word processing and keeping references. Students undertaking a taught Masters will usually have training built into their programme, whilst prospective PhDs will usually have to undertake a certain quota of 'research training modules' before they can progress to the latter stages of their degree. MDs, which are expected to be part of a higher professional training, are often the least well supported with formal training modules, so it is worth ensuring that you attend a research methods module and some IT coaching, if you are heading for an MD but are underconfident in these at the start. Such modules/master classes are run both regionally by academic or NHS R&D units, or by national organizations such as the Royal College of General Practitioners, who will advertise forthcoming events in their journal and website.

Having got yourself into the general 'system', your other practical problems can be summarized as '3M': *Mentoring, Mindset,* and *Method.* All these relate to core process

features, especially important in original research programmes over a long period. The whole point of doing a
higher degree is to gain a mental *training*. Many find it fun,
but no-one finds it easy. Therefore you need to take supervision and support very seriously, develop the attitudes
that will see you through, and be systematic and rigorous
from the start.

Mentoring

Mentoring refers to the role of the nominated academic
supervisor and other expert resources, but also to peers
who are doing or have done the same thing, and to the
general support you could get from your family and
friends. On a taught masters you may well be allocated a
tutor, but with original research you yourself must identify someone within the institution of your registration
who has expertise in the field you have chosen, and
someone who you feel will both challenge and support
you. A graduate studies tutor may help to find the right
person, but you should always meet a prospective supervisor and agree that you can probably work together. Use
these early contacts to clarify issues such as frequency of
supervision, means of contact, long-term availability, and
expectations. Then, identify a 'research buddy' who can
talk you through the research process as a peer, and
whose work schedule may parallel your own. Finally,
make sure your domestic and work partners have some
idea of the demands and activities involved, so that they
can support you as needed. Going to research seminars
and workshops can also be a valuable way of gaining
expertise and support.

Mindset

While good mentoring and support can make a lot of difference, having the right mindsets will be very important to your progress. Research is a self-directed and isolated business; it does not leap up and hug you, nor get on quietly without you. It is emotionally neutral, but will reflect like a mirror your moods and frustrations. Data collection and analysis often is slow work, with many setbacks and problems. Literature searching and writing up are often overwhelming as one fights to structure a seemingly unending pile of paper into logical and decisive output. You will also need a remarkable amount of time alone with your work, in order to be rigorous and thorough; the mental mindset of research cannot be created in 5 minute spaces. Remember it is a *training*: in gaining new skills, pursuing trains of thought, in problem solving, in reflection and critical thinking, and in developing conceptual understanding. This is a marathon: you run it alone, over a long period, and some bits are harder than others.

Methods

This refers, not to the research methods for the study, but to the crucial importance of being organized throughout your work. You need to develop clear physical systems for retrieving articles, data, and preliminary analyses: those crucial field notes may be illegible 12 months on, and 20 unlabelled floppy disks with unlabelled SPSS charts equally wasteful of your time and efforts. Research participants will become disenchanted if you fail to arrive at the time stated to do a data collection, or forget half your equipment. Think through the implications of each stage before you dive into the action: be methodical. Others who have done higher degrees themselves may be the most useful source of training here.

During the degree: a model for experiential learning

Although education and training may be interpreted as provision by others, higher degrees are a quintessential model for self-directed adult learning. The typical research student is responsible for locating and updating the background literature, for making choices about appropriate methods to answer the question asked, for carrying out data collection in an ethical and honest way, for rigorous analysis, and for not wasting public money or time by leaving data unanalysed and unpublished. The supervisor's role in this training is intellectual criticism, retaining the overview of the thesis, and a degree of guidance in resources and skills. It is also to

. . . .supervise

To look them over

To look beyond

With my farseeing eye

An eye that looks back

Remembering the cloud of confusion

Hypothesis and hype

'I can I can't

Too much too hard

Too onerous

On call was never like this, it

Never ends.

I have created a monster'[9]

The principles of adult learning[10] are therefore relevant here. Briefly, these are that:

- participants are not usually in full-time education;
- process accommodates and acknowledges varying needs and backgrounds of participants;
- draws on experience and skills of participants;
- assumes motivation ('need to know');
- assumes competence ('can learn', 'can learn how to learn');
- utilizes reflection to create learning from experience;
- respects autonomy;
- role of supervisor is facilitative not didactic.

Thus those who undertake a higher degree must be keen independent learners and be prepared to analyse and overcome their own weaknesses.

The outcomes—education and training for others

When your degree is complete, the NHS then has a new individual who is trained in the use of research methods and rigorous intellectual training. Apart from the outcomes mentioned earlier, it is likely (indeed, appropriate) that those who have undertaken higher degrees help to train others. This may be through writings, workshops, taking on teaching or supervisory roles, and by disseminating skills to one's own working context. You can drive your practice team mad by asking them to define the aims and objectives of the practice meeting; amuse your friends by asking them for the evidence base behind their condemnation of the Health Authority's latest cutbacks; and rise to fame by confounding local consultants at a CME meeting with your erudite debate informed by your own work! In spite of the escalating number of GP[3] and nursing higher degrees,[11] there is still a very low critical mass of primary care practitioners with an academic perspective, so the new graduates are immensely valuable in the dissemination of a research-oriented culture. And a PhD is after all a way to have more doctors on the team!

Some examples

This final section describes some fictionalized health workers who are all in a position to consider doing a higher degree. These case studies are based on real people, are included to help you consider whether your perspective resembles any of these characters, and to consider some factors that can be taken into account when deciding whether the model of a higher degree is the best means of training for meeting your needs. They also show some ways in which such decisions can influence, and be influenced by, colleagues within the same organization, thus demonstrating that the ability to undertake a higher degree does not usually come only from the individual concerned. In the current environment where practices must be more proactive to meet the education and training needs of the team, higher degrees will inevitably be an option which most teams will at some point be asked to consider for suitable members of staff. They are certainly an option which can be very beneficial to practice over a career lifetime.

Dr Tom Cluny

Dr Cluny did general medicine for 3 years as an SHO before completing a vocational training 5 years ago. He is a GP trainer, the PCG clinical governance lead, an active member of the RCGP, and has done several courses on evidence-based practice. He is keen to progress to an associate adviser position, but decides that first he will undertake an MD into the reasons why GPs do not always comply with evidence-based protocols. He registers at his old medical school, does a refresher course in research methods at the local academic unit, communicates with his supervisor largely by e-mail, and carries out the field work while maintaining his current post. He negotiates a 6-month study leave based on 'Red Book' money to write up his thesis, and at the end of this time seeks and obtains an Associate Adviser post.

Comment

This is a very self-motivated person who had been persuaded of the value of an MD while still in hospital practice. He espouses some traditional forms of an academic GP (RCGP, higher degree, academic appointment in postgraduate general practice) but uses his skills largely in the GP community and does not want to reduce his practice commitments.

Ms Ellen Russell

Ms Russell is the practice nurse. She originally did an English degree at Oxford University, then did her nursing qualification as a mature student, and is now a mother of three school-age children. She is a keen folksinger and musician. Within the practice, she has always been a leader of innovations in health promotion, favouring talking therapies over medication. She is critical of the contemporary NHS competence-driven culture, but has recently been active in an MRC trial on back pain, and is the lead on new approaches to chronic obstructive airways disease in which she is now an accredited trainer. Dr Cluny suggests that, given her academic ability and leadership potential, she might get a lot out of joining the local multidisciplinary Masters in Medical Science course on a part time basis over 3 years, for which the practice could release her.

Comment

This colleague certainly appears able, but she decides she has no reason to undertake such a prolonged further academic training. She feels no need to prove herself academically, and prefers to be led by the needs of the practice and her own creativity.

Mr Chris Marsh, CPN

Chris really enjoyed his specialist mental health training, and having practised for 3 years is now keen to extend his skills. He is bright, extrovert, and eclectic: wants to train other people but also gain more skills himself. He has kept up his reading and knows that there is a lack of local expertise in proven cognitive approaches to enduring mental illness and phobias. He is nervous of pushing himself towards becoming a trainer, or of asking for study leave, but brings up the possibility of further training at his annual appraisal. His line manager is keen to keep Chris on the staff, and suggests the Trust might support him to undertake a local Masters course (MSc in psychological therapies). Chris is shocked: all his mates tease him about the idea. Nevertheless he applies, is accepted, based on his nursing training, and in spite of some initial difficulties getting to grips with the work thoroughly enjoys himself. His practical skills work in therapy are excellent, but his grades are average, largely due to lack of prior similar experiences of writing and analysing ideas. Nevertheless, with some firm supervision he graduates, and immediately expands both the skills of the team and his own practice, while now being eligible to become a sector team leader.

Comment

Chris is an example of someone who had no sense of themselves as a potential academic, and needs encouragement and opportunities put in his way by a well-informed senior colleague, to the benefit of the Trust and the service.

Mrs Janet Redfern

Janet is the health visitor. She and Dr Cluny have both been active participants in the local research practice network, and she has been instrumental in securing research funding for the practice to carry out various studies. Her husband, an orthopaedic surgeon and himself an MD, has now been offered a 2-year posting to Bahrain. He is keen to take this, and their children are just the right age to live abroad without losing substantial schooling. However, Janet is concerned at a further service break, knowing that Bahrain will be a difficult environment for her to be clinically employed. Since both she and her husband are forever discussing work, and she has always had a good critical mind, they decide that she could plan towards a PhD for which she could work while they live away. She and Dr Cluny seek funding for a comparative study of breast-feeding practices in the UK and the Middle East, for which she finds supervisors in both settings.

Based in part on this work, Janet gains her PhD and the practice is accredited as a level 2 RCGP research practice, thus further enhancing their track record and making more funding likely.

Comment

Academic work can be compatible with family life, and research-active members in a practice can make a major contribution to future income and status.

Dr Ann Howell

Dr Howell is an enthusiastic clinician, and has always led on undergraduate teaching in the practice since she first became a partner. She works six sessions a week, but now that her younger child is entering school she is considering further work. One of her colleagues tells her that the university department of general practice are looking for someone to become a part time lecturer (1 day a week) to resource problem-based teaching groups with the final year students. At the interview panel the Professor asks her: 'have you ever thought of doing a higher degree?' Her honest answer is 'no' . 'Why not?' 'No-one ever told me I could do that as a GP.' Going home, she muses on how she has never been given any role model of an academic GP. Within 4 years she has completed her MD while still working as a GP, and with this qualification is in a position to apply for a full-time academic post. From here she becomes a well-known academic, active for the profession at a national level. People even ask her to write book chapters about the role of higher degrees in primary care.

Comment

Be warned—doing a higher degree can change your life!

References

1. Look MJ. Institutional sources of medical school faculty and patterns of personnel flow among medical schools. *Academic Medicine* 1998; **73**: 77–83.
2. Pincus HA, Haviland MG, Dial TH, Hendryx MS. The relationship of postdoctoral research training to current research activities of faculty in academic departments of psychiatry. *American Journal of Psychiatry* 1995; **152**(4): 596–601.
3. Williams WO. A survey of doctorates by thesis among general practitioners in the British Isles from 1973 to 1988. *British Journal of General Practice* 1990; **40**: 491–4.
4. Calvert G, Britten N. The UMDS MSc in general practice: attainment of intended outcomes. *British Journal of General Practice* 1998; **48**(436): 1765–8.
5. Boex JR, Boll A, Franzini L, *et al.* Understanding the value added to clinical care by educational activities. *Academic Medicine* 1999; **74**: 1080–6.
6. Howe A, Avery A, Carter YH. Evaluating higher degrees from general practice—case not yet proven? *Education for General Practice* 2000; **11**(2): 150–6.
7. Calvert G, Britten N. The UMDS/St Thomas's MSc in general practice: graduate perspectives. *Medical Education* 1999; **33**(2): 130–5.
8. Mant D. *National Working Group on R & D in Primary Care: Final Report.* London: NHS Executive, 1997.
9. Howe A. In: 'Afterword'. *Undertaking Higher Research Degrees: Some Practical Guidance.* London: RCGP Research Group, 2000: 30.
10. Brookfield S. *Understanding and Facilitating Adult Learning.* Milton Keynes: Open University Press, 1986.
11. Pelletier D, Donohugue J, Duffield C, *et al.* The impact of graduate education on the career paths of nurses. *Australian Journal of Advanced Nursing* 1998; **15**(3): 23–30.

Further reading

Howe A, Carter Y, Thomas K, Green F. *Undertaking Higher Research Degrees: Some Practical Guidance.* London: RCGP Research Group, 2000. (This booklet is available free of charge from the Royal College of General Practitioners.)
Carter YH, Thomas CP, eds. *Research Opportunities in Primary Care.* Oxford: Radcliffe Medical Press, 1999.
Burton JL. Get a Masters degree in education. *BMJ Classified* 8/1/2000; 2.

13 Educational interface between primary and secondary care

MICHAEL BANNON AND
ELISABETH PAICE

Introduction: the primary secondary care interface

The international primary care movement may trace its more recent origins from the pivotal conference held at Alma Ata, USSR, in 1978, where it was determined that the goal of achieving the best possible results in health gain for the world's population by the year 2000 should be met through the platform of primary health care.[1] Subsequently, many countries have endorsed the objectives set at Alma Ata by means of effecting a shift in emphasis, with primary rather than secondary care being the main focus in health-care delivery. In addition, more attention is now devoted towards activities that promote healthy lifestyles and disease prevention. With respect to the NHS, change in this respect has been driven by successive reforms, which has led to the development of GP fundholding in the 1990s and more recently, the emergence of primary care groups and primary care trusts. Prior to these developments, a three-tier service was in place with the majority of patients receiving health care from GPs and other members of the primary health care team, a minority requiring the services of local district general hospitals, and a much smaller number still being referred to highly specialized, tertiary services. In addition, boundaries between these services were strictly demarcated in terms of management, accountability, and budgetary control.

All this has changed. The majority of chronic illness is now managed at primary care level. For example, more than 95% of mental illness is managed in the community[2] and care for the majority of patients with diabetes has also shifted from hospital settings to general practice.[3] In a similar fashion, a significant amount of health promotional activity, including child health surveillance,[4] is now within the remit of primary care.

Changes in the balance between primary and secondary care are now evident (Figure 13.1). This has of necessity resulted in new configurations of staff working in both primary and secondary care. Health professionals now work in other settings in addition to those traditionally associated with their perceived roles. Hospital specialists now undertake outreach clinics in primary care and some GPs work as clinical assistants in hospitals. Changing skills are evolving with staff developing new areas of competence and expertise and extension of existing ones. The term 'primary secondary care interface' has been used repeatedly in both published papers and discussion documents that have considered this evolving situation.[5] We could identify no precise and widely agreed definition of the term. From a pragmatic point of view the primary secondary care interface might be considered as a point in health-care delivery where:

- professionals from primary and secondary care work more closely together;
- traditional boundaries are blurred and move flexibly to best meet the needs of patients;

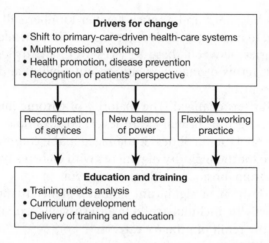

Figure 13.1   The balance between primary and secondary care.

- skills, knowledge, and experience are shared;
- roles may be extended and be transferable.

Such is the perceived importance of the interface that there are at least 50 recent publications in peer-reviewed journals which describe various aspects of the concept. There is, in addition, a website, constructed by the Department of Health, which is devoted to the subject (http://www.doh.gov.uk/ntrd/rd/psi/). The site provides details of research that has been commissioned by the NHS Executive, in the first instance around 21 priority areas relevant to the primary secondary care interface which have the following general themes:
Outpatient services:

- referrals (appropriateness, cost-effectiveness);
- view of patients, GPs and specialists;
- outreach clinics undertaken by specialists in primary care settings.

Transfer of services out of secondary care:

- chronic disease management;
- extended roles of nurses both within primary and secondary care.

Guidelines:

- development and evaluation of guidelines;
- prescribing.

Background and principles of education and training in primary and secondary care

Whilst the above developments will result in both new training needs and demands for a variety of training methodologies, it must not be forgotten that much has already been achieved in the training of professionals working in both primary and secondary care. Both under-graduate and postgraduate medical education and training were previously delivered primarily in the hospital setting. In the past this made sense, since hospitals were where facilities, clinical teachers, and patients were to be found. However, the nature of general practice has changed dramatically over the last 50 years. Group practices are now increasingly common, operating from purpose-built premises and employing a comprehensive variety of health-care professionals. The primary care setting has become both practical and appropriate for an increasing range of educational activities. Whereas most of the education of doctors still takes place in hospitals, a range of initiatives to move education to community settings including primary care have been successfully implemented. We explore some of these here in detail, and consider why this move is desirable and how far further it should be encouraged in the future. In doing so, we endeavour to keep in mind some principles that we feel should guide those encouraging such a move:

- Doctors (and other health professionals) should be prepared for the conditions in which they will practise by being educated in settings that reflect those conditions.
- Health professionals need to understand every aspect of the journey their patients may have to take through the health-care system.
- Exposure to practice in less popular specialties and underserved communities will hopefully encourage some doctors to work in those settings.
- The quality of education and clinical supervision must be assured whatever the setting in which it is delivered.
- All professionals work most effectively as part of functioning teams. They must appreciate and respect each other's role in the delivery of health care to patients.

What do different clinical settings have to offer for education and training?

Teaching hospitals

Whilst it is generally agreed that teaching hospitals have held the monopoly of medical education for too long, it is worth remembering the unique opportunities they offer. They tend to be large and based in urban areas, with the widest range of tertiary services. They have sicker, more complex patients who spend more time in hospital and are therefore more readily available for the teaching of physical signs. Teaching hospital out-patient clinics are often specialized, offering concentrated exposure to a narrow range of problems. They also offer efficiencies in the concentration of patients, teachers, and researchers, as well as physical facilities such as libraries and seminar rooms. On the other hand, senior staff have to cope with a variety of pressures. Research, administration, and other non-clinical responsibilities can have an impact on their involvement in teaching or training. The latter may be delegated to senior trainees, sometimes to mutual benefit, but sometimes not. The concentration of students and junior doctors may lead to competition for clinical experience. Increasingly, teaching hospitals deal with cases that may be too ill or complex to use for teaching; length of stay is shorter; pre- and post-operative care is out of hospital; out-patient clinics are closing and patients are being followed up in their local district general hospital or GP practice.

District general hospitals

For the last 10–20 years, the role of district general hospitals in offering medical education and training at every level has been growing, and there are now few without placements for undergraduate and postgraduate doctors at every level. These hospitals tend to be busy, sited in cities or large towns and dealing with more common, less complex cases than teaching hospitals. There are fewer medical staff, and these are more likely to be directly involved in delivering the service. Each district general hospital has its postgraduate centre, library services, and programme of educational activity. Some have well-developed links with local practices and encourage GPs to share educational facilities. However, considerations of cost and patient preference have reduced in-patient stays, and led to increasing development of day-case surgery.

At the same time, reductions in junior doctors' hours and total training time have left these hospitals even more short of medical staff, so that there is little spare capacity for teaching and training.

Primary care

The primary care setting offers the opportunity to encounter patients with undifferentiated problems; the ability to observe the natural history of diseases, and to observe or provide care over time; the everyday relevance of integrating preventative strategies into care plans; and the immediacy of social and behavioural issues in patient care.[6] The community setting allows the student to learn to recognize and treat common complaints, evaluate and manage chronic illness, incorporate health promotion and disease prevention into their practice, appreciate the community and cultural context of illness, and educate and counsel patients about their illness.[7] In this setting, however, the student or trainee will see a significant proportion of patients with ill-defined signs and symptoms that never add up to a diagnosis. Well managed, this experience will help put secondary and tertiary care into perspective. Poorly managed, it may lead to frustration, disillusionment or diagnostic nihilism. Other disadvantages are the low concentration of patients with specific conditions; lack of continuity when patients are referred to secondary or tertiary care providers; relative lack of experience of trainers; and isolation from other learners. Finally, training in the general practice setting is costly.

Educational principles

Whatever the setting, the same educational principles apply. Each placement should have defined educational objectives and the wherewithal to achieve those objectives. This must include an appropriate case mix to provide necessary clinical experience. An induction procedure should be in place, which includes introductions to key members of staff, a timetable, an outline of the responsibilities of the post, and unambiguous guidance about whom to contact when in need of help. The supervision should be appropriate to the experience of the learner, who should rarely feel forced to cope alone with problems beyond his or her competence, but should be encouraged to take graduated responsibility. Some time should be set aside each week for teaching, as well as group or individual discussion with a supervisor. All teachers and trainers should be prepared for and supported in their role. If it is not possible to achieve these principles in a community setting, then training should take place in a hospital setting, but with explicit attention to conditions in the community.

What do different settings offer at different stages?

Undergraduate teaching

The bulk of undergraduate clinical teaching has traditionally been carried out in the secondary or tertiary care setting. The arguments for continuing this arrangement include the concentration of clinical teachers who are leaders in their field and engaged in research; the convenience of having students on one site for lectures, tutorials, and group work; the efficiency of providing library and information services. The disadvantages include inculcating the attitude that most health care is properly delivered in the hospital setting and that a career in hospital medicine is more desirable than one in the community. Evidence that this happens is well documented in Simon Sinclair's study of the factors that influence the attitudes of medical students.[8] There has been increasing emphasis on primary care in the undergraduate curriculum. More clinical placements are now in primary care and aspects of the curriculum, such as clinical skills, have been taught in that setting. Has the initiative been successful? In a recent study, GPs who taught clinical skills were asked about the effect of teaching and teacher training on their morale, confidence in clinical and teaching skills, and clinical practice. The main theme that emerged was a positive effect on morale. This was attributed to peer and professional support; improved teaching skills; revision of clinical knowledge and skills; a broadening of horizons; contact with enthusiastic students; increased time with patients; improved clinical practice; improved teaching skills; and an improved image of the practice. Problems with teaching were due to external factors such as lack of time and space and anxieties about adequacy of clinical cover while teaching.[9]

The pre-registration year

The pre-registration year was introduced over 50 years ago in order to ensure that recently qualified doctors could not go out into independent general practice without a year of working under supervision in hospital. Since then there have been many reports questioning the educational quality and relevance of the year. Teaching hospital posts are traditionally highly sought after, largely because of the perceived value of the references to be gained, but the house officer has little opportunity to take responsibility and may end up inundated with routine tasks of little educational value. The district general hospital is likely to offer more challenge, but may ask too much of recent graduates. Certainly stress levels amongst house officers in both kinds of hospital posts are high.[10]

General practice, with its record of taking training seriously, has much to offer the pre-registration house officer. Referrals to hospital involve complex decision making, in which the house officer can take part. The house officer will have the opportunity to reflect with patients and their families how referral impacts on the individual and their family. They will learn that patients in primary care have a high degree of autonomy, which requires a different style of clinical disease management. They will recognize that it is essential for the doctor to form a bond of understanding with the patient and work with the patient to achieve cooperation and success.[11] They will be exposed to professional relationships within the multidisciplinary health-care team, and learn the mutual respect that should exist between the medical profession in the primary and secondary care sectors.

General practice has been included in the pre-registration year at St Mary's Hospital, Paddington, for over 10 years,[12] but this initiative had not been widely adopted until 1998, when the General Medical Council recommended more pre-registration posts in general practice.[13] Funding was made available to postgraduate deans to develop 4-month postings in general practice as part of 1-year rotations including 4 months each of general medicine and general surgery. Evaluation of the first of these new schemes revealed that the clinical experience available was considerable[14] and satisfaction with the training at least as good as in traditional posts. Stress levels in trainees completing a 1-year rotation were lower than in those completing a pair of traditional 6-month hospital posts.[15]

However, in implementing GP pre-registration house officer (PRHO) posts, there are various practical issues which need to be given careful consideration. The recurring presence of an inexperienced doctor in a training practice for a 4-month period can be disruptive and labour intensive for the practice. It is important to balance the needs of PRHOs with the interests and safety of patients. Certain patient groups, for example, very young children, require special consideration due to the relative inexperience of PRHOs. Unaccompanied domiciliary visits to patients can pose a problem for similar reasons. PRHOs in general practice are at risk of feeling isolated, and need to meet their peers. This could be achieved by integrating PRHOs into the local vocational training scheme or it may be more appropriate to establish a local support group for PRHOs, run on similar lines, with appropriate course organizer input and financial support.[16]

Career aspirations and factors influencing them

One of the reasons given for including general practice in the pre-registration year is to encourage recruitment.[17] At a time when the NHS is determined to develop a primary-care-led service, we are seriously short of GPs. Although nearly 40% of doctors are needed to work in general practice, many make the choice late, after failing in, or becoming disillusioned with, a career in a hospital specialty. Predominant exposure to specialist clinical role models who teach within tertiary care hospitals moves people away from family medicine.[18] Young doctors working in a hospital setting are likely to be encouraged by their

A general practice suitable for PRHO training should:

- include at least two principals, one of whom should be nominated as the educational supervisor;
- have a close working relationship with the university's general practice department or unit;
- be within easy reach of the medical school or a post-graduate centre;
- offer a wide range of primary health-care services;
- have ready access to laboratory services, radiology departments, and an adequate library.

The PRHO must:

- always have available a senior doctor to provide assistance;
- have a clinical workload which allows time for further education;
- be resident either in a hospital approved for general clinical training which is conveniently near to the health centre or in the area served by the practice and within easy reach of the health centre.

GMC[13]

consultants to follow in their footsteps, and attitudes to a career in general practice are often negative, as evidenced by these quotes by PRHOs:

On leaving my job my consultant voiced concern that I might be bored and wasted by pursuing a career as a GP. It made me angry, but upset too.

My consultant surgeon refused to accept I would be anything but a surgeon.

There have been swings in the attractiveness of general practice as a career in the past, which have been related to levels of remuneration and the nature of the general practice contract. Whether increasing the exposure of young doctors to work in primary care will encourage more to choose general practice as a career may depend on the enthusiasm expressed by their teachers. If what they are exposed to is a demoralized and disillusioned supervisor, the effect may be quite the reverse.

The SHO grade

Specific training for doctors to become GPs was first implemented in the 1970s. The scheme that was finally accepted (the vocational training scheme) comprised 2 years' experience in a variety of approved senior house officer (SHO) posts in hospital, coupled with 1 year in general practice. The appropriateness of hospital posts in the vocational training of GPs has been questioned, but plans to base training in general practice with secondment to hospital for short periods of carefully selected experience would have dramatic consequences for the hospital service.

The principal complaints of trainees, course organizers, and trainers in general practice are that the hospital component is not relevant to the needs of GPs; teaching is poor and irregular; study leave is difficult to obtain; and the duration of posts is too long.[19] Considerable efforts have gone into improving the training and conditions of work of SHOs. Regular surveys of trainees can pinpoint problem areas and direct attention to those areas in most need of change. A survey in North Thames in 1996/7[20] showed that 52% of 1316 SHO respondents rated their posts good or excellent. The major exception was in obstetrics and gynaecology where only 31% of SHOs considered their posts good or excellent. Further analysis revealed that it was the intended GPs in obstetrics and gynaecology who were particularly dissatisfied (Figures 13.2 and 13.3).

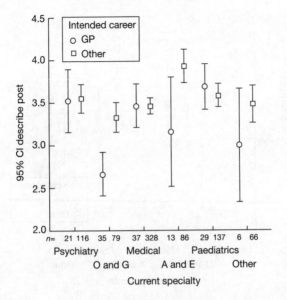

Figure 13.2 Satisfaction with SHO training posts—North Thames, 1996/97. Responses to the question: 'How would you describe your post to a friend who was thinking of applying for it?' Responses were on a scale of 1–5 where 1 = very poor and 5 = excellent, and are presented as mean scores with 95% confidence intervals.

They differed from their specialty orientated colleagues in being less likely to have discussed their objectives with a consultant at the beginning of the post; less likely to have had feedback on their performance; less likely to have had a useful induction to the post; and less likely to be satisfied with the clinical experience they were acquiring. These posts were all reviewed by the deans of postgraduate general practice education, and recommendations made to consultants about appropriate induction, feedback, supervision, and relevant educational opportunities. Two years later, when the survey was repeated, improvement

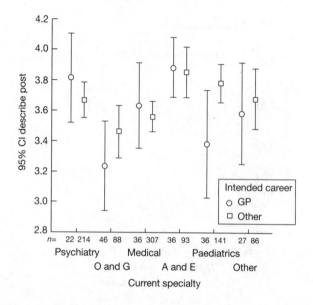

Figure 13.3 Satisfaction with SHO training posts—North Thames, 1998/99. Responses to the question: 'How would you describe your post to a friend who was thinking of applying for it?' Responses were on a scale of 1–5 where 1 = very poor and 5 = excellent, and are presented as mean scores with 95% confidence intervals.

had occurred to the point where was no significant difference between the ratings given by intended GPs and career SHOs.

Whilst there are undoubted problems in providing appropriate experience in the hospital setting, there are also limitations to the opportunities offered by practice-based learning. Good jobs as an SHO are an asset to any registrar in general practice. Patients seen in hospital are often more sick than those whom GPs treat at home or in a cottage hospital. The ability to distinguish between a seriously ill child and a child who is merely upset is probably one of the most valuable lessons learned during a hospital paediatrics attachment.

Taking primary care education into the secondary care setting

A number of surveys in different countries have shown that patients attending emergency departments often have problems that could more appropriately have been dealt with by a GP. Primary care patients need a primary care response, but staff in A&E departments often lack training in identifying and responding to the broad range of physical, social, and psychological problems that present in this setting. A scheme for bringing primary care education to accident and emergency SHOs has been successfully implemented in at least one unit and may prove a useful model.

Changes to GP Training

In April 2000, it was agreed that the budget for GP vocational training would move from the General Medical Services budget to the Medical and Dental Education Levy (MADEL). This shift will lead to new opportunities for doctors training to be GPs. These will include the opportunity to spend a larger part of the training in primary care pursuing a particular learning need, such as learning about the management of drug addiction. The new arrangements will allow the directors of postgraduate general practice education to provide more opportunities for refresher training for doctors returning to general practice and for those who have trained abroad. Despite the different regulatory arrangements for England and Wales, Scotland, and Northern Ireland, there has been close liaison between directors and all health departments. This means that these new opportunities will be available across the UK depending on local needs.[21]

Information technology support in education and training in primary care

Flexible and changeable working patterns across the interface between primary and secondary care are highly dependent upon comprehensive recording and transfer of information. Until now, the main basis for recording information consisted of hospital and GP case notes. Communication largely consisted of letters and telephone calls between interested parties. The potential contribution of computerized information technology has been recognized. The demand for rapid information transfer has led to the development of electronic patient records, data links with hospital pathology systems, and the use of clinical guidelines with decision support software which have been embedded in GPs' computer systems. There is also scope for the expansion of telemedicine which will enable consultations between primary care staff and hospital-based specialists.[22] Two educational aspects with respect to information technology need consideration. Many staff, particularly those working in secondary care, may require further training in clinical information systems. Second, educational opportunities are inherent in the electronic dispersal of protocols and guidelines.

Future educational and training needs across the interface

Recognition of the importance of the primary secondary care interface will undoubtedly result in further training needs for professionals, which are currently unmet. These educational needs may be in part predictable, but further research across all professional groups working at the interface could well yield interesting results.

Altered service configuration with rapid shifts in the traditional balance of power will inevitably result in confusion, anxiety and feelings of loss on the part of many professionals, especially those currently working mainly in secondary care. GPs, because of the nature of their training, may well possess an advantage in this respect. The 2 years of hospital SHO posts that most GPs complete as part of vocational training provides them with an insight into the challenges and idiosyncrasies of working within secondary care. On the other hand, hospital specialists, to date, have rarely worked outside secondary care. As a result, their understanding of the primary care within the new NHS is likely to be impaired. There is both anecdotal and published evidence of negative perceptions on the part of hospital doctors toward their colleagues in primary care. One such study among A&E house officers revealed disturbingly negative perceptions about general practice.[23] Furthermore, qualitative research reveals much confusion and misconceptions upon the part of both GPs and specialists regarding their respective roles, responsibilities and power.[24] It follows that educators in all disciplines will face a considerable challenge with respect to positively influencing attitudes. A core curriculum for all professionals who work across the interface is required with the ultimate aim of removing barriers and altering traditional professional boundaries and mind sets (see Box 13.2 for suggestions). Clinical staff will need to be aware of the current shift in emphasis away from secondary care. Attention should be devoted to the whole issue of role definition and appreciation. It follows that much needs to be done with respect to ensuring that professionals know about the roles of others and that they are able to work with others as part of teams with clearly defined roles.[25] The NHS Plan strongly advocates the principle of 'substitution' whereby professionals, usually nurses, will undertake some of the roles traditionally played by others in an attempt to break down barriers and remove lines of demarcation.[26] Again, this concept will result in more challenges for providers of education.

How might this be achieved?

Challenging but exciting times lie ahead for educators. From experience so far, it would seem that at least the following should be considered in the very near future:

- Training need analysis of all professional groups at all levels (undergraduate, postgraduate, established practitioners) should be undertaken in order to determine the current awareness and future skill needs associated with working at the interface.
- In the case of secondary care specialists, some consideration should be given to including within their training some structured exposure to general practice. For example, one paediatric department in northwest London ensures that specialist registrars in that speciality have the option of doing a clinic per week in a local GP surgery. It may also be possible for GP principals to work in hospital clinics or A&E departments with the same objective in mind.

Box 13.2 Suggested curriculum of training for professionals working at the primary secondary care interface

How the NHS is changing

- Shifting emphasis from secondary to primary care
- Multiprofessional working
- Increasing accountability
- Incorporating views of patients

Systems and system failures in the NHS

- Planning a service across organizational boundaries
- Clinical guidelines: development, implementation, and evaluation
- Clinical effectiveness
- Clinical risk and its management

Role appreciation

- Defining roles
- Transferring roles
- Extending roles

Referral

- How and when to refer to other professionals
- Safe handover
- Recognizing own limits

Flexibility

- Working in different settings
- Development of new skills
- Innovation in practice
- Coping with ambiguity and uncertainty

- Cooperation is needed with respect to deaneries, universities, confederations, and primary care groups in order to ensure that the principles of multiprofessional working including role awareness, are included in training at all levels.

- As a starting point, the Clinical Effectiveness Project could act as a focus for existing professionals who currently work at the interface.[27] This process requires professionals of all disciplines to focus upon a clinical area of common interest, to agree upon the most effective way of delivering a service to patients and to explore resources, skills, and training needed in order to achieve agreed objectives.

The concept of the primary secondary care interface offers an important focus for the education of all healthcare professionals, but especially doctors, who have tended to function well on either side of the interface but not so successfully across it. The problems faced at the interface are of prime importance to the patient, and it is here that the young doctor can best learn the importance of effective communication, teamwork, and systems, as well as the value of considering every aspect of the care they offer from the patient's point of view.

References

1. Mahler H. The meaning of 'Health for All by 2000'. *World Health Forum* 1981; **2**: 5–22.
2. Gask L, Sibbald B, Creed F. Evaluating models of working at the interface between mental health services and primary care. *British Journal of Psychiatry* 1997; **170**: 6–11.
3. Pierce M, Agarwal G, Ridout D. A survey of diabetes care in general practice in England and Wales. *British Journal of General Practice* 2000; **50**: 542–5.
4. Hall DB. Purchasing of community child health services—how and how much (work in progress).

5. Hausman D, Le Grand J. Incentives and health policy: primary and secondary care in the British National Health Service. *Social Sciences Medicine* 1999; **49**(10): 1299–307.

6. Saunders NA. Specialist training in community settings: an educator's perspective. Canberra Policy Forum, 20 November 2000.

7. Shipengrover JA, James PA. Measuring instructional quality in community-orientated medical education: looking into the black box. *Medical Education* 1999; **33**: 846–53.

8. Sinclair S. *Making Doctors: an Institutional Apprenticeship*. Oxford: Berg, 1997.

9. Hartley S, Macfarlane F, Gantley M, Murray E. Influence on general practitioners of teaching undergraduates: qualitative study of London general practitioner teachers. *British Medical Journal* 1999; **319**: 1168–71.

10. Firth-Cozens J. Emotional distress in junior house officers. *British Medical Journal* 1987; **295**: 533–6.

11. Hayden J. Why PRHOs in General Practice? In: Paice E, ed. *Delivering the New Doctor*. Edinburgh: ASME Medical Education Booklet, 1998.

12. Wilton J. Pre-registration house officers in general practice. *British Medical Journal* 1995; **310**: 369–72.

13. General Medical Council. *The New Doctor*. London: GMC, 1998.

14. Cohen M. The GP preregistration house officer: the potential learning experience of primary care. *Hospital Medicine* 1998; **59**(6): 502–4.

15. Firth-Cozens J, Moss F, Rayner C, Paice E. The effect of 1 year rotations on stress in preregistration house officers. *Hospital Medicine* 2000; **61**(12): 859–60.

16. Jackson N. General practice in the pre-registration year: barriers and practical considerations. In: Paice E, ed. *Delivering the New Doctor*. Edinburgh: ASME Medical Education Booklet, 1998.

17. Morrison JM, Murray TS. Career preferences of medical students: influence of a new 4 week attachment in general practice. *British Journal of General Practice* 1996; **46**: 721–5.

18. Tepper J. Internal schisms are bad medicine. *Canadian Family Physician* 1999; **45**: 558–9.

19. Bayley TJ. Commentary. The hospital component of vocational training for general practice. *British Medical Journal* 1994; **308**: 1339–40.

20. Paice E, Aitken M, Cowan G, Heard S. Trainee satisfaction before and after the Calman reforms of specialist training: questionnaire survey. *British Medical Journal* 2000; **320**: 832–6.

21. Field S. Career focus. Vocational training for general practice. *British Medical Journal* 2000; **321**: 2.

22. Reardon T. Handbook of telemedicine. *Telemedicine Journal* 1999; **5**(3): 315–16.

23. Dale J, Williams S. Attitudes towards general practice and primary care: a survey of senior house officers in accident and emergency. *Journal of Accident and Emergency Medicine* 1999; **16**(1): 39–42.

24. Bowling A, Redfern J. The process of outpatient referral and care: the experiences and views of patients, their general practitioners, and specialists. *British Journal of General Practice* 2000; **50**(451): 116–20.

25. Finch J. Interprofessional education and team working: a view form the education providers. *British Medical Journal* 2000; **321**: 1138–40.
26. Department of Health. *The NHS Plan: a Plan for Investment, a Plan for Reform.* London: DoH, 2000.
27. Adams C. Clinical effectiveness: a practical guide . . . a six-part bi-monthly practical guide to clinical effectiveness. *Community Practitioner* 1999; **72**(5): 125–7.

14 Mentoring in education and training

ROSSLYNNE FREEMAN

Introduction

This chapter begins with a distinction between the two activities of training and education which influence the take up of the mentor's role. The traditional role of a mentor is described, then compared with the role of modern mentors in nursing, education, and medicine to consider what this might tell us about the role of mentors in primary care settings. The requisite skills and knowledge base for mentors is placed within the context of education, before finally considering the potential for tasks for mentors in primary care.

Distinguishing education from training

Considering the potential role of mentors in the new world of primary care begins with recognizing the distinction between education and training. Training is a process of acquiring skills to carry out a specified task, with a clearly observed outcome—like a clinical protocol. We train people through sustained repeated structures of showing them how, supervising them whilst they practise how, and, when we judge their ability to follow the procedures and produce the required outcome sufficient, we leave them to it. From this is derived familiar maxims—practice makes perfect, see one, do one, teach one.

Education appears as a broader, more complex task. In the process of introducing new knowledge, it widens horizons of understanding beyond the teaching of a single subject, incorporating possibilities of explanation outside the familiar and the known. Those who proudly tell us that they 'have been to the university of life' are grasping at this concept of broad knowledge gained in diverse ways. Education is less concerned with the direct *application* of knowledge gained, more concerned with equipping individuals to retrieve knowledge and apply it accurately and relevantly when faced with events and dilemmas in professional life, and to know how to search out new knowledge when critical gaps in 'knowing' appear. Training shows us the known, education prepares us for the unknown (Box 14.1).

Separating the two activities does not imply that there is no overlap. It is generally accepted that people being trained to perform a particular function will learn quicker and more efficiently if they understand the context of that function, why it is performed as it is. In this way we see the acquisition of knowledge, and understanding of it,

---

Box 14.1

Training

Acquiring skills for a specified task with a known outcome

Education

Preparation for the unknown: retrieving knowledge to respond accurately to complex problems

directly applied to the task—an integration of knowing why, learning how, and knowing when.

Overlapping examples of training and education abound in medicine, most particularly in general practice. The GP 'Trainer' (paradoxically a task owing much more to education than training) works with their Registrar, an adult professional, already trained and skilled in the profession of medicine—but requiring their knowledge to be focused and applied in a particular context. When trainers speak of the challenge of their training role, the challenge described lies not in terms of *training* their Registrar to become a competent operator of various clinical procedures, but in terms of *educating* them in the art of family medicine, inculcating attitudes and behaviours appropriate for family medicine. This education includes encouraging the Registrar to develop insight into self and patients, recognizing how their own doctor behaviour influences the outcome of the consultation, how their attitudes influence other members of the primary care team. It is 'whole person' teaching, infinitely more complex than training, infinitely more challenging, and, by the same token, a process infinitely more rewarding in its execution.

Implicit in this last example is the concept of 'holism'. One outcome of traditional medical training is that it leads some doctors to see not a patient in front of them, but a manifestation of disease. Increasingly, medical training is placed within the community which it serves, moving medicine back to the holistic values embodied in the Hippocratic oath, which held together science and art, and encouraged compassionate medical practice which perceived the patient in the context of their family, their working life, community, and culture. Recent imposed changes in primary care in the NHS have focused on 'putting the patient first'—urging primary care groups towards structures which, at best, provide a service responsive to the needs of their community, rather than the needs of the health professionals.

Similarly, adult education embodies the concept of holism. Friere[1] argued that the learner must be seen within the whole context of their lives, and through his work illuminated the inter-relationship between the student, their environment, and the ultimate application of their new learning which empowered them as change agents in their communities. Hence knowledge is power— but, it seems, most powerful when acquired in ways that acknowledge the student as a whole person, whose learning is subjected to the constraints and opportunities that surround their daily life.

Learning in adulthood then became associated with teachers who do not simply impart nuggets of wisdom, leaving the student to memorize it, regurgitate it whole at examinations, and then promptly forget it, but teachers who consider the person in front of them, and how they might relate to them in ways which maximize their opportunity to learn not only new knowledge and skills, but something about themselves as people, encouraging personal development. This is the basis of humanist education currently popular in primary care settings—spawning the language of self-directed learning, learner-centred programmes, learning communities, and, not least of these, the role of the teacher as a facilitator of learning. From this we begin to discern the link between the values of professional adult education, and the values that underpin the role and function of mentors, for they too are concerned with facilitating learning in ways that develop the person professionally and personally. To determine this connection more clearly, let us revisit the role and function ascribed to the original Mentor.

Mentoring past and present

Before considering the classic role of a mentor and its relevance to primary care, let me ask you, the reader, at this point, to pause in your reading, and answer this question: 'Can I identify a mentor in my own life?' If your answer to the question is 'yes', you might like now to consider the particular qualities that this person possessed, and reflect on why you perceive them as a mentor—why do you ascribe the name 'mentor' rather than friend, or colleague?

If you have answered 'no' to the question, and could not locate a meeting with a mentor in your life thus far, you are probably wondering why—and even whether it says something about you! If so, it might be helpful to remember that mentors—effective, 'true' mentors—are few and far between, and we are fortunate indeed if, at some stage of our professional journey, we encounter one, and experience a mentoring relationship. Whilst effective mentoring spontaneously occurs for some, enlarging the possibilities of chance through more overt professional support structures would benefit more people. It is precisely this realization that underpins the development of mentoring projects in medicine today.

Mentors are associated with the classic Homeric concept of a mentor as faithful friend and guardian, wise teacher, and counsellor. In Homer's Odyssey,[2] Odysseus (Ulysses), King of Ithaca, asked his wise and faithful companion, Mentor, to oversee the upbringing of his young son Telemachus whilst he, Odysseus, went off to fight the Trojan wars. Mentor was asked to guide Telemachus from childhood into adulthood, instilling values and attitudes that would prepare him for his future role as king. True to politicians then and now, Odysseus predicted a fast and decisive victory for himself and his army—another war to end all wars. But the fighting, together with a number of unforeseen delaying strategies employed by the gods, led to his continuing absence over 20 years. Eventually, tired of waiting, and growing more angry at the behaviour of the suitors besieging his lonely mother, Telemachus set out to search for him. Mentor accompanied him on his journey, supporting and guiding him when critical choices had to be made. At the end of the journey, Telemachus had matured both inwardly in spirit, and outwardly, in being able to manage life events and function independently.

This is the familiar, known aspect of the Greek story which inspires the vision of a mentor—a wise, yet neutral companion, who objectively observes the obstacles and hurdles that litter the path of the journey towards maturity and independence, offers suggestions and support for surmounting them, gives critical feedback on outcomes, is kindly and encouraging, yet ultimately stands apart from the action. When the journey is accomplished, the mentor departs.

Central to the story of Mentor, and reflected in the fairy stories of other cultures that came later, is the concept of *transition*. The characters (with whom we all identify) face numerous obstacles that have to be overcome in order to achieve the desired goal—aggressive dragons prevent access to the sleeping princess, and have to be slain. Other beautiful princesses have to summon up the courage to kiss repellent frogs to find their ideal life partner. From time to time, along the way, another person—often in various guises—appears, and offers advice or suggestions as to how best to proceed. The message is always that the journey, which demands that we develop tactics for surmounting these obstacles, and the nature of our relationship with the people who alight on our path as the journey is undertaken, is more important than arriving. In the journey a transition is made from uncertainty and dependency, to more confident maturity, with independent thought and action. When we arrive, we realize how influential was this person who appeared at just the right moment, it seems, to ensure that we stayed the course and moved forward.

Perusing the story closely, one sees that Mentor made little distinction between Telemachus the boy—as he then was—and the future Telemachus who would become king. In social psychology this is the present and future self–entwined.

It is this hidden dimension of the tale which precisely describes the essential task of mentoring, and how it is distinguished from other forms of intervention, such as educational supervision. It is the mentor's role and task to facilitate and support an individual to make transitions—from where, and who they are now (the present self)—to what they might become (the future self).

Modern mentors

Box 14.2

The essential task of today's mentor remains the same as that of the traditional Homeric mentor—to facilitate an individual in his or her transitional journey from where, and who, they are now, to what they might become.

Has this essential ability of the original Mentor been lost in translation into today's market place? How would we now describe the role and function of a mentor? Definitions are so wide and various that Merriam[3] concludes that mentoring is defined by context—institutions and organizations define a mentor role so as to meet their own particular organizational needs. There are, for example, primary care groups who have delegated the task of helping individual practitioners to prepare and implement personal development plans to people whom they call 'mentors'—thus defining the mentor's role as being related to a particular activity necessary to the organization. Philips-Jones[4] opts for a straightforward statement that mentors are 'influential people who help you reach life goals'. A review of mentoring in six organizations by the Incomes Data Services saw mentoring as a process that facilitates the transfer of skills and experience between different levels of staff.[5] Other authors attach less importance to the influence and seniority of the mentor, and more to their skill in facilitating personal and professional growth. Taking an overview of definitions of mentoring from a range of professions and disciplines led to the introduction of mentoring in general practice using the following description of mentoring, one which seeks to uphold the opportunity for transitional work:

A mentor is a senior practitioner, or respected peer, who offers, through the medium of an ongoing professional relationship with his/her mentee, opportunities to maintain, develop, and stimulate their professional development. They do so through addressing current concerns and identifying learning needs, providing space and time to reflect on, and evaluate professional practice. The mentor identifies blocks or hindrances to the professional well-being of their mentee, offering help and support for the mentee's personal and professional development.[6] (page 47)

So fashionable is the term 'mentor' today that it encompasses a myriad of tasks and functions under the general umbrella of staff development. For this reason, it is perhaps more helpful to consider not the range of definitions of the task, but some of the distinctive attributes that separate mentoring from other forms of intervention—such as appraisal, or educational supervision. These will include the following.

The nature of the relationship

The relationship should be equal, dynamic, and to a great extent voluntary. The mentoring relationship should be one of equality—the mentor does not exercise personal or organizational power through imposing hierarchical status, but strives instead to empower their mentee through their skilled facilitation.

The relationship between mentor and mentee should not be too comfortable, which risks collusion and stagnation, but dynamic, ever-changing, containing constructive challenge alongside support.

Mentoring is ideally a voluntary activity, for when mentoring is enforced, it runs the constant risk of being perceived as a disguise for performance appraisal, or some assessment of competence—the iron fist in the velvet glove.

The mentee-directed nature of the work

It is for the mentee to think about, and come prepared to present their mentor with the agenda they want to address. It is the mentor's task to set aside any personal agendas of their own, in order to pay full and unbiased attention to the current issues, interest, and concerns of their mentee. This reflects again the dynamic nature of mentoring, which is not a passive activity. The mentee needs to 'do their homework' beforehand, and the mentor needs to respond actively

Continuity

Mentoring is not a one-off meeting, like annual appraisal, nor is it a social conversation. It is a continuing relationship, over time, until both parties decree that the mentoring work has been addressed, and the mentee moves on. Most mentoring relationships have a natural time span, but mentors are responsible for reviewing and summarizing the working agenda, ensuring that it stays focused and purposeful.

Mutual gains

Whilst the mentor is directed towards supporting and developing their mentee, this does not exclude their own professional development, which comes from the mutual regard, and shared learning, of their mentoring relationships, and from their own continuing mentor education and support.

Mentors in education, nursing, and medicine

Although mentoring is a new innovation for professional development in medicine, the disciplines of education and nursing have long experience of mentorship. Their related, but different, application of the mentor's role provides us with a sharper illustration of the earlier distinction made between 'training' and 'education'.

Nursing has issues akin to those of medicine. It has a tradition of learning through the apprenticeship model, and today faces similar demands for practitioners to be accountable for their continuing education and professional development. As in medicine, this demand has led to the development of mentoring programmes that owe rather less to altruistic desire and more to political expediency. A further similarity is existing confusion over terminology. Whilst Morle[7] wryly points out that the absence of a clear definition of the role, function, and preparation of a mentor has not hindered take-up of the idea, and shares with other authors concerns that the 'bottom up' approach to mentoring relies on an informality that too easily slides into mentoring systems that lack clear description, objectives, and a measure of accountability.

Looking at the dominant models of mentoring in the nursing profession implies that for the most part mentoring was associated with training, rather than education.

When the apprenticeship system pertains, as it does in one form or another in every profession, mentoring is first and foremost seen as a craft model—an experienced practitioner supporting the young practitioner as they make the transition from apprenticeship to mastering their craft and thereby gain admittance to the professional group. Parallels can be drawn here with general practice trainers, or practice managers taking on a new member of the primary care team. New entrants into the craft guild of primary care need not only training in necessary skills—such as communication in the doctor–patient consultation, or managing an appointment system—but inculcating into the customs, rituals, and beliefs of the practice group. Training for the task sits alongside acculturation into the organization.

The roles and skills of the mentors are then associated with training practitioners—teaching skills, supervising clinical procedures, setting up training programmes and writing protocols, overseeing the acquisition of skills, and providing feedback as practitioners moved through various stages of training. And from nursing comes another term relevant to mentor roles in primary care—the term 'preceptor'.

The preceptor's role is clearly tied to clinical practice, but encapsulates a feature of mentoring which nursing pays much more overt attention to than other professions—that of role modelling, as is made clear by this definition of preceptorship by Chickerella and Lutz as:[8]

(preceptorship is) an individualised teaching/learning method in which each student is assigned a preceptor so that they can experience daily practise with a role model, a resource immediately available within the clinical setting.

Here we see an important focus on role modelling through supervised clinical practice, a more 'hands on' position than that of our original Mentor who stood back, allowing his student to develop in autonomous ways. Burnard and Armitage[9] make a clear distinction, seeing the role of a preceptor as being:

more clinically active and more of a role model than the mentor. The preceptor is more concerned with the teaching and learning aspects of the relationship, whilst the mentor, although concerned with these things, seeks a closer and more personal relationship. (page 226)

This is a view supported by Morton-Cooper and Palmer[10] but they also go on to consider the overlap between training activities and learning support. Before considering mentoring as applied to education, it is worthwhile pausing to recall that at times, alongside his objective, supportive partnership to 'educate' Telemachas towards his future role as king, Mentor was not remiss in the occasional 'hands on' training of his young mentee.

In summary, the main features of mentoring undertaken within the context of training emerge as ones which are short term, and focused to support the new entrant into the profession, providing supervision, feedback on mastery of the task, learning support, and offering a role model for good practice. Are these features replicated when mentoring in educational settings is explored?

Yes—to some extent. But in higher education, we find a broader range of mentoring interventions, moving more towards the educational concept of assisting experienced professionals to work with the unknown, developing skills and knowledge which enable them to both resolve, and contain, the unexpected outcomes in professional life. Mentoring in education adapts to the professional 'age and stage' of the mentee, emphasizing the self-directedness of the mentee and the continuity of the mentoring relationship. Thus, mentoring is perceived as a relationship which goes beyond the apprenticeship state—for example, inducting new teachers into the profession—to becoming a means of staff development.

As illustration, consider the example of a university teacher who, during her appraisal, identified with her appraiser a career goal of moving into a more senior research post within the following 2 years. Her appraiser advised working with a mentor to develop knowledge and skills in team leadership, foreseeing that a more senior role would demand skills in team management which this teacher did not yet possess. In the mentoring relationship, her mentor encouraged her to reflect on her present relationship with peers—her communication styles, 'critical incidents'—those events that had produced positive or negative outcomes with colleagues—her responses to challenges from her students, and how she managed the group dynamics when engaged in small group teaching. Examining her *present* knowledge and skills helped this mentee to forecast *future* skills. With her mentor, she could identify areas for attention and further development—which prepared her for being asked in interview how she might cope with taking on a team management role.

This moves the education model closer to medical models. Kelly *et al.*[11] see mentoring as an effective means by which newly appointed educational leaders—head teachers, faculty heads in universities—can explore with a mentor the organizational aspects of their appointment—the structure and systems of their new organization and the underlying values existing within it, and the individual strengths and weaknesses that influence the execution of their role. In this way, the mentor provides support directed towards their becoming more quickly and effectively established in their leadership role.

Here we see the wider original Homeric dimension of exploring the present-and-future self held intact. The themes that have emerged from the work of mentors in medicine show that they, too, have been encouraging practitioners across the whole range of professional life— new entrants to the profession anxiously finding their feet, established practitioners running out of enthusiasm after years in the job, those about to take on a new role— to take stock of their present self, and then to plan the next stage in the journey towards their future self, overcoming obstacles such as conflict with partners, managing boundaries between personal and professional life, coping with the stress of change, setting manageable goals for a future career.

This concept of on-going mentoring builds in two related features that characterize it as educational rather than training. First, evidence from educational and psychological literature suggests that individuals are more likely to set themselves targets and change their behaviour as a result of feedback from a peer than from a line manager. This supports the earlier contention that mentoring is a relationship of equals, but the second related feature is that, when mentors are assigned throughout the hierarchy, more practitioners have the experience of both giving and receiving mentoring, and this in itself builds a supportive structure throughout the organization. In nursing, role modelling was an important feature of mentoring. In education, perhaps the most important dimension is that of offering some measure of personal support. Here the interface between the personal and the professional self is openly acknowledged, and included as a primary source of mentoring work. The need for the mentor to nurture their mentee in both their personal and professional development is more overtly stated.

Yet both professions have long documented the difficulties encountered when, alongside giving personal support, the mentor role has included an assessing function. This highlights the potential for mistrust in the mentoring relationship. If in the context of 'personal support' a mentee makes a disclosure to their mentor, what reassurance do they have that such information would not be used in judgement against them? If the relationship is non-hierarchical, and confidential, then the mentee relies on their own assessment of the trustworthiness of their mentor, evidenced in the mentor's presentation and management of the mentoring relationship, and the overall credibility of the mentor scheme. However, if it is hierarchical (and many so-called mentoring relationships exist between senior managers and junior employees) and the boundaries of confidentiality are not clearly stated, then it could be safely assumed that sensible mentees would filter the information they gave to their mentor. This is particularly so if the mentor has some influence on, or control over, their future career.

Observing the potential conflict between 'supportive mentor' and 'reporting appraiser' reported by other professions, it would be reasonable to conclude that this is best avoided by separating the two roles entirely. For those of you reading this chapter with a view to setting up a mentor framework in your organization, the author would urge you towards this course of action!

At other times, roles are inherited whereby the policing function and pastoral care sit side by side. However, anyone who has ever been drawn into a close personal relationship with someone whom they then have to sack from the management team, or confront with evidence of their perceived failure in achieving a task, will recognize how the lessening of social distance diminishes the ability to act dispassionately. Trainers in general practice tell of their difficulties when they have befriended their Registrar, and, later in their relationship, have had misgivings about signing them up as competent to undertake independent practice. It requires that the mentor has to walk the tightrope between their own and their mentee's personal and professional self more cautiously. This leads Black and Booth[12] towards a radical view for *excluding* the personal dimension of mentorship, based on their view that no learning gains were made if the mentoring relationship was over-supportive, collusive, and non-critical. More reasoned views support the importance of the mentor having defined skills and knowledge which enable them to combine personal support with constructive challenge (Box 14.3), thus avoiding collusion and inappropriate support.

Box 14.3

If mentors are to be effective facilitators of professional development, they need to offer not only warm encouragement and empathic support, but appropriate challenge and confrontation.

This is the grit in the oyster that will move the mentee forward—and further.

In summary, it is not surprising to find that education offers a model of mentoring which reflects the concepts of education rather than of training. When applied to young entrants to the profession, the transition from apprentice-teacher to membership of the profession focuses on the application of new theoretical knowledge to the concrete experience of taking up the professional role—the theory-to-practice exercise which includes the personal dimension—'how are you responding to this?' As practitioners become more established, and take up new roles, mentoring is focused on integrating past knowledge and experience with new, untried, untested roles—'where have you been and what will you now become?' Here we see a longer-term intervention, with a wider dimension, one which explores unknown and uncertain territories to develop strategies for surviving the unexpected outcomes in professional life. In this way, mentoring in the context of education moves the practitioner more towards rigorous *self*-appraisal, and away from the *other*-appraisal common to training.

Skills in mentoring

Exploring the models of mentoring in training and education shows that mentoring takes place at different levels. The skills of the mentor are matched to the level of their intervention, and the context in which it takes place. This is not to imply value judgements on levels, but to recognize that the longer-term interventions that have been described above will require the mentor to have skills that go beyond first-level facilitation, to developed insight and intuition with which to assist their mentee in their transitional journey. Egan's[13] basic ingredients of a skilled helper begin with the necessity of good communication, both verbal and non-verbal, listening empathetically, offering positive acceptance to the other, being non-judgmental. These skills encourage the mentoring relationship through its stages:

- creating the appropriate climate, with trust and good communication between mentor and mentee;
- reflection on practice and review of professional life, identifying learning needs;
- giving constructive feedback on professional issues;
- developing strategies for coping with change;
- enhancing understanding of situations and their position in it;
- setting goals and monitoring development.

Mentors are seen as people who facilitate this process. But what does 'facilitation' mean?

Being a facilitator is, like apple pie and grandmothers, generally perceived as nurturing. The word conjures up all things honourable—smoothing the way for events to happen, making difficult 'things' easier. Like the word mentor, 'facilitator' is increasingly used as an umbrella word in medical management, yet the role of a facilitator is rarely described, they have no job description beyond being facilitative. The NHS appoints 'facilitators' who are called in to practice groups and departments usually in times of trouble, bringing with them the expectation that they will help sort things out and bring about resolution, or at least lessening, of the current conflict or dilemma. The skills for achieving this are commonly associated with those described earlier, together with effective small group leadership. At its most dangerous, facilitation is undertaken by individuals who, for whatever reason (not all bad), assume that if they create a warm climate in a group, and do a few introductory exercises so that people start talking to each other in a friendly and supportive way, the rest will take care of itself. They have completed the task of 'facilitating', and the responsibility for on-going work and outcomes is then handed over to the group.

This suggests a partial, incomplete interpretation of the word 'facilitator', one which is certainly insufficient for mentoring. Creating a trusting climate and promoting dialogue is certainly a necessary and essential first stage, but the facilitator's work has only just begun. Education provides a more expanded view of the facilitator's role, more akin to skilled mentoring. Brookfield[14] points out that it is all too easy to see the job of a facilitator as one concerned solely with assisting adults to meet those educational needs and professional aims which they themselves perceive and express as meaningful and important. This is a flawed, if comfortable, perception of an uncomfortable task, for facilitation has much more to do with confrontation and challenge than support and reassurance. A true facilitator points out the contradictions in a learning plan, or a statement made, confronts an individual with their own conflicting behaviours, is capable of suggesting more complex alternatives, and can prompt critical reflection on an action. Facilitators painfully and uncomfortably scrutinize assumptions on which statements and actions are based, they question the values that underpin behaviour, and generally make a nuisance of themselves. The skills defined as necessary for this unpopular role include negotiation, constructive confrontation, and appropriate, well-timed challenges to the status quo, and problem solving. They are drawn down from a number of different theories and disciplines—most particularly from management, psychology, education, and counselling—to provide the mentor with a sound knowledge base from which to develop a range of skills with which to assist their mentee's professional journey, whether they be at the first stage of apprenticeship, or established practitioners seeking self-development.

A final word on mentoring skills. It is generally accepted that the most effective mentors are those who have themselves undergone a transitional journey, who understand the experience of forging ahead down diverging paths littered with obstacles that have to be overcome. This will have enabled them to develop insight into their own personal and professional selves, making it more possible to promote that in others. But if mentors are to realize this and other benefits that accrue to them through the privilege of performing the mentor role, then they, as mentors, in their own turn, will need continuing education for, and support in, undertaking the work of acting as a mentor.

Notwithstanding the requisite skills of mentoring, how might they potentially be applied in the new scenarios of primary care?

Mentoring in primary care

This chapter has discussed how the essential transitional task of mentoring can be embodied in contemporary mentoring, and how education rather than training embraces the characteristics of a mentoring role. Now we turn to some speculation on the potential tasks for mentors in primary care settings.

Surviving constant change

The process of change has fascinated authors and researchers from all disciplines, and produced general agreement that the stages of change encompass an initial period of shock and denial—'this can't be happening'—

followed by a period of destabilization and general choas when familiar coping strategies become overwhelmed by the force of change. Usually this is followed by a gradual acceptance of the new order, and attempts to adapt to it. Caplan[15] points out that a critical factor in the successful coming to terms with a new order is the availability of support—people, like mentors, who can offer consistent and available support to individuals as they move through the change process. The more overt the support structure, the better the prognosis for successful adaptation. Fink[16] describes how organizations also react initially with defensiveness, going through stages of angry acting-out behaviours, before accepting the inevitable and turning their energies towards getting the best out of the new situation. Staff support, he concludes, is an important factor for organizational survival.

Destabilization is heightened when the change includes the merging of previously distinct groups. The recent spate of mergers of hospital trusts have highlighted only too clearly the natural tendency of individuals and groups within organizations to guard their territories fiercely, and fight to retain 'their' operational ground. Similar responses are found in primary care groups, where members from the merging general practices eye each other warily over the conference table, attempting to assess each other's defensive capabilities. Little wonder that facilitators of 'away-day' events for newly formed primary care groups have enjoyed a boom year, as members of the disparate groups attempt to find common ground, a collective identity which will unite them under a single banner.

Leadership

In this transitional process the ground is staked out, and positions are taken up. Individuals and groups alike seek out allies with whom to plot strategies which will bring them their desired piece of action, the requisite power to enable them to influence the future, and realize visions and ambitions. This opening scene ushers in the various leadership bids. Some individuals actively seek leadership positions, keen to become major players in the new order. These new leaders may be motivated by *retaining* power— hence the traditional view that the leadership positions will be occupied by doctors 'because they always have been'—or conversely by *claiming* power with which to announce their entry into the new arena as key protago- nists rather than supporting players. Other members of the group, perceived by their colleagues as 'natural' leaders, find the role thrust upon them. Others find lead- ership thrust upon them because no-one else appears to want to wear that particular crown. And then there are those who observe the bidding process from a distance, perhaps reflecting on their previous experience which taught them that leadership is all too often a poisoned chalice.

It would seem that Telemachus had similar misgivings about his leadership role more than once, and had it not been for Mentor might have given up kingly ventures and gone home to his mother. But we know that he did not, mainly because his mentor stayed alongside him during the change process, helping him reflect on experience, plan some further coping strategies, and then provided feedback for him on their implementation.

Exactly the same role exists for today's mentors in primary care. Fisher and Cooper[17] write of anticipatory transition, when one thinks oneself into future roles so that appropriate attitudes and behaviour patterns can be rehearsed before the transition occurs. Mentors in primary care can work alongside those anticipating the take-up of a new role, acting as sounding boards for hopes and ideas, envisioning likely problems, identifying areas of strength. Newly appointed leaders, as we learn from the professions of education and nursing, benefit from being supported through the process of change when the previous role is relinquished, and the new one explored, tried on, adapted to fit the wearer.

Multidisciplinary working

The period of destabilization in the change process is more acute when groups are grappling not only to overcome the intergroup barriers that prevent the formation of a collective identity, but also to break down interdisciplinary barriers. Multidisciplinary working challenges the basic assumptions we make about other professional groups. It is the nature of group life to consider one's own professional group superior to others. We enter into the hugely enjoyable pastime of denigrating other professional groups, because this serves to strengthen our bonds of professional kinship and supremacy. Faced with a new order which insists that all professionals in the primary care team are equals, we outwardly change our behaviour to accord with this principle, whilst inwardly reflecting that some are more equal than others. To move away from the familiar assumptions and stereotypes that have served our professional bonding needs so well, for so long, is to risk yet further destabilization. What if we find that, after all, social workers do not all wear sandals, read the Guardian, and can never make a decision, or that you can no longer confidently predict that every surgeon you meet will be male, sexist, a rigid thinker, and arrogant into the bargain? As Breakwell[18] infers from her work on identity, testing assumptions about other groups rocks the stability of your own, as dialogue reveals assumptions that other professionals have made about you.

Here we find another important role for a mentor in primary care, for one immediate route for crossing boundaries is to work with a mentor from outside your own profession. The real test of the mentor's worth lies in their application of skills and knowledge, and their ability to interpret their role. For example, a GP mentor was assigned to a psychologist who was finding himself struggling to maintain a constructive relationship with the supervisor of his PhD thesis. The psychologist asked to work with a mentor outside his own profession who would offer a neutral and objective perspective on an interpersonal problem. The mentor, from his 'outsider' position, yet using his skills of compassionate enquiry married with constructive confrontation, was able to explore with his psychologist-mentee the assumptions that the mentee had made about himself, including his self-doubts about his intellectual ability. These doubts continually surfaced when he contemplated discussing openly and honestly with his supervisor the difficulties in their relationship, and prevented him from speaking out. The mentee felt further inhibited by complex issues of ethnicity and cultural values that lay between them. The mentor's exploration of these themes, followed by his continuing support whilst the mentee developed strategies for discussing the issues directly with his supervisor, enabled the mentee to manage a series of difficult encounters with his supervisor. Finally, the mentee concluded that although he had initially assumed that the tension in the supervisory relationship stemmed entirely from his own intellectual ignorance and failure to understand, his supervisor was not without his own difficulties and shortcomings when it came to organizing his own thinking, and the subsequent demands he made upon his students.

The mentee thereafter swiftly and successfully negotiated with his university a change of supervisor, even though this was not normal practice and cost the university extra money, and went on to successfully and happily complete his thesis. The mentor remained in almost total ignorance of the subtle dimensions of psychology, and their relationship to his mentee's thesis, but, notwithstanding, occupied his mentor role confidently, employing his skills and knowledge to good effect.

This example demonstrates that it is not always necessary, or indeed desirable, that mentor and mentee share the same professional role. Rather, their objectivity and outsider status could be used to challenge the ready assumptions made between same-professionals, to seek clarification and rationalization rather than allow statements to go untested. Mentor himself, remember, did not occupy the same royal role and status as his mentee, but acted as external mentor, testing assumptions and gently challenging 'known' truths.

Organizational benefits

Mentoring across professional boundaries, whilst being an individual activity, inevitably contributes positively towards establishing professional dialogues between different disciplines, which in their turn aid the group's collective identity.

We can begin to see the possibilities opening up that individual mentoring can produce benefits not only for the mentor and their mentee, but for the organizational group as a whole. To illustrate, consider some recently imposed change—the requirement that all members of the primary care team have personal development plans (PDPs), which are written expressions of an individual's present and future potential. These individual statements have to be matched to the overall future potential of the organizational group—the Practice Development Plan, incorporating the aims and objectives of the primary care team. This, in turn has to relate to the government's own health agenda.

If this enforced change is to 'succeed'—in the sense that it achieves positive and lasting organizational benefits— the implementation of developmental plans require interested scrutiny, followed by consistent monitoring and review—an activity which typifies learning communities. All too frequently a plan for change is formulated, implemented, and then left to run itself. Thus, it is insufficient to prepare a PDP, sign it, then consign it to a filing cabinet to be pulled out a year later at the next round of staff appraisals. The action plans agreed within the statement —be they plans for further learning, reorganizing, or developing a new service to patients, undertaking an audit— need to be discussed and reviewed, amended in the light of new or unforeseen developments, and compared with the progress of the Practice Development Plan. Here the mentor's consistent role makes them available to monitor the individual implementation of PDPs, to encourage the primary care team to plan when and where review meetings should take place, and act as coordinator of individual aims with organizational objectives.

Role change

Sometimes development plans include taking on new roles, discussed earlier in terms of leadership roles. But changing roles is not a simple business—it is complex, and often uncomfortable. Karasek[19] perceives increased levels of stress when the job holder previously enjoyed a high degree of personal latitude in decision making, and now finds autonomy lessened and accountability to others heightened. Taking up a new role, as Telemachus discovered, means balancing out personal desires with the expectations and demands of others.

John Spencer, in an earlier chapter, refers to the tension between educational development and performance management. A similar tension exists when managing roles. All professionals enjoy, to a greater or lesser extent, the ability to interpret their role according to personal perceptions, but these have to be set alongside the terms of the contract and the job description. When change occurs, as it has in the NHS, some practitioners are left unable to comfortably fit their personal values and beliefs about how a job should be carried out, with the values and beliefs exhibited by the organization. The content of mentoring work in general practice showed the confusion and disillusion suffered by doctors who saw the central tenents of general practice—continuity of care, the unique nature of the doctor–patient relationship—eroded by changes imposed via government edicts.[6] This illustrated the misfit between the doctors perception of their role, and the changed demands and expectations of the NHS. In primary care, the mentor's task is to find ways in which the differing perspectives of a role can be reconciled, a creative intervention enabling health professionals to work within the changed order with a reasonable degree of enthusiasm and a continuing sense of commitment.

Conflict

Whilst role change can bring transient conflict, more persistent is conflict between team members. Here, the neutrality and objectivity of the mentoring relationship can enable the mentee to trace not only the source of interpersonal conflict, but see their own contribution to it—difficult this, as naturally we believe ourselves to be in the right. The mentor, standing apart from the agendas, and acting without judgement, is in a good position to explore with their mentee how their own attitudes and behaviours may influence the conflict, and develop strategies which, if not resolving the issue (many interpersonal conflicts cannot be totally resolved), may enable the mentee to manage it more effectively and reduce damage to themselves.

Here again is organizational benefit, for reducing levels of interpersonal conflict within groups not only enhances the well-being of the individual, but releases energy for the collective task.

Isolation

In education, and other professions, those at the top of the organization have mentor support. This is in recognition that those who occupy leadership positions or senior management roles may find themselves isolated, cut off from support structures previously accessible, as has happened in primary care. Fortunate managers find like-minded souls in primary care groups elsewhere, entering into an informal co-mentoring relationship in which each person supports the other, talking through their experiences, and seeking feedback and ideas for management. If that opportunity does not easily present itself, their isolation maintains. Similarly, at the other end of the scale, people occupying roles which have been thrust upon them, or who find that a role voluntarily sought now overwhelms them, need support to survive, to find the precarious balance referred to earlier between personal satisfaction and organizational demand. Protected time for *all* team members, high flyers and strugglers included, to reflect on experience and receive some constructive feedback on role management, is a further use of mentoring within the primary care scene.

Celebration

In newly formed organizations, mentors are associated with struggle. Individuals struggle to create a new identity in a changed order, the organization itself struggles to establish a strong and collective identity for the group. In this context we could easily overlook findings that show mentors are about empowerment—enabling individuals to take charge of their professional life, not merely survive it. Their very existence in an organization declares a commitment to a working environment that encourages creative practice and discovers learning that benefits individuals and team alike. We can celebrate the achievement that mentoring has already to brought to the profession of medicine, and confidently anticipate the yet-to-be discovered element that the practice of mentoring in primary care will add to the mentor's tale.

References

1. Friere P. *Pedagogy of the Oppressed*. Harmondsworth: Penguin, 1969.
2. Translation of Homer, *The Odyssey*. See, for example *The Odyssey*. New York: Simon and Shuster, 1969.
3. Merriam S. *Mentors and Protégés: a Critical Review of the Literature*. Adult Education, San Francisco, Jossey-Bass, 1993.
4. Philips-Jones L. *Mentors and Protégés*. New York: Arbour House, 1982.
5. *Income Data Study*. 1996, Study 613.
6. Freeman R. *Mentoring in General Practice*. Oxford: Butterworth-Heinemann, 1998.
7. Morle KMP. Mentorship—is it a case of the Emperor's new clothes? *Nurse Education Today* 1990; **10**: 66–9.
8. Chickerella BG, Lutz WJ. Professional Nurturance—preceptorships for undergraduate nursing. *American Journal of Nursing* 1981; **81**(1): 18–117.
9. Armitage P, Burnard P. Mentors or preceptors—narrowing the theory practice gap. *Nurse Education Today* 1991; **11**: 225–9.
10. Morton-Cooper A, Palmer A. *Mentoring and Preceptorship*. Oxford: Blackwell Science, 1993.

11. Kelly M, Beck T, Thomas J. Mentoring as staff development. In: Wilkin M, ed. *Mentoring in Schools*. London: Kogan Page, 1992.
12. Black D, Booth M. Structured mentoring. In: Wilkin M, ed. *Mentoring in Schools*. London: Kogan Page, 1992.
13. Egan G. *The Skilled Helper—a Systematic Approach to Effective Helping*, 4th edn. Pacific Grove, CA: Brooks/Cole, 1990.
14. Brookfield SD. *Understanding and Facilitating Adult Learning*. Milton Keynes: Open University Press, 1996.
15. Caplan G. *An Approach to Community Health*. London: Social Science Paperbacks, 1969.
16. Fink S, Beak J, and Taddeo K. Organisational crisis and change. *Journal of Applied Behavioural Science* 1971; **7**: 15–41.
17. Fisher S, Cooper L. *On the Move: the Psychology of Change and Transition*. Chichester: Wiley, 1990.
18. Breakwell G. *Coping with Threatened Identities*. London and New York: Methuen, 1986.
19. Karasek RA. Job demands, job decision latitude and mental strain. *Administrative Science Quarterly* 1979; No. 24.

Acknowledgement

The author is grateful to Dr. Elizabeth Sullivan, Senior Research Fellow at De Montfort University for her illumination of the concept of present and future self in the context of mentorship.

Index